Coronaviruses

(Volume 1)

Edited by

Jean-Marc Sabatier

Institute of NeuroPhysiopathology
Marseille, Cedex
France

Coronaviruses

Volume # 1

Editor: Jean-Marc Sabatier

ISBN (Online): 978-9-81149-896-1

ISBN (Print): 978-9-81149-894-7

ISBN (Paperback): 978-9-81149-895-4

need for a court order if at any point you breach any terms of this License Agreement. In no event will any delay or failure by Bentham Science Publishers in enforcing your compliance with this License Agreement constitute a waiver of any of its rights.

3. You acknowledge that you have read this License Agreement, and agree to be bound by its terms and conditions. To the extent that any other terms and conditions presented on any website of Bentham Science Publishers conflict with, or are inconsistent with, the terms and conditions set out in this License Agreement, you acknowledge that the terms and conditions set out in this License Agreement shall prevail.

Bentham Science Publishers Ltd.
Executive Suite Y - 2
PO Box 7917, Saif Zone
Sharjah, U.A.E.
Email: subscriptions@benthamscience.net

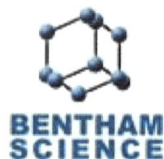

BENTHAM SCIENCE

CONTENTS

PREFACE

In this difficult period of the SARS-CoV-2 (and its variants) infection responsible for Covid-19 diseases, the importance of scientific works and reviews dealing with these viruses has never been more essential and vital. This book brings together essential data regarding prevention (vaccination), detection, and various approaches (chemotherapeutic drugs and antibodies) to the potential treatment of coronavirus infections. It consists of six chapters concerning, (1) the effect of candidate drugs chloroquine and hydroxychloroquine on QT interval in infected patients with Covid-19 diseases (chapter 1 by Aleem *et al.*), (2) the impact of the Covid-19 pandemic for the South Asian Association for Regional Cooperation (SAARC), comprising the Bangladesh, Bhutan, Maldives, Nepal, Pakistan, Sri Lanka, India, and Afghanistan (Chapter 2 by Kanwar *et al.*), (3) the humoral immune response in humans based on anti-SARS-CoV-2 antibodies to treat Covid-19 diseases (chapter 3 by Çalık1 *et al.*), (4) the antiviral potential of herbal-based immunomodulators (chapter 4 by Kumari *et al.*), (5) the various methods and strategies for diagnosing SARS-CoV-2 (and its variants) infection in hosts/humans (Chapter 5 by Narvekar *et al.*), and (6) the resistance to the spread of SARS-CoV-2 and related Covid-19 diseases within a population based on the pre-existing immunity of a high proportion of individuals as a result infection or previous vaccination (chapter 6 by Tiwari & Sahu). Such a book comprising a compilation of key data on SARS-CoV-2 and Covid-19 should certainly be a tool of crucial importance for researchers around the world working on these research themes, as well as for clinicians confronted to a growing number of patients with Covid-19 (data from 20th April 2021: 141 million cases of SARS-CoV-2 infection worldwide, with over 3 million deaths).

Jean-Marc Sabatier
Institute of NeuroPhysiopathology
Marseille, Cedex
France

List of Contributors

Abdul Aleem	Internal Medicine, Lehigh Valley Hospital, Allentown, PA, USA
Aditya Narvekar	Department of Pharmaceutical Sciences and Technology, Institute of Chemical Technology, Mumbai-400019, India
Ameya Chaudhari	Department of Biomedical Engineering, Duke University, Durham, North Carolina-27708, USA
Amit Kumar	Department of Chemistry and Center of Advanced Studies in Chemistry, Panjab University, Chandigarh, U.T.-160014, India
Anita Venaik	Department of General Management, Amity Business School, Amity University Noida Uttar Pradesh– 201313, India
Betül Mutlu	Yıldız Technical University, Faculty of Chemical and Metallurgical Engineering, Department of Bioengineering, Istanbul, Turkey
Bhargawi Mishra	Department of Neurology, Institute of Medical Sciences, Banaras Hindu University Uttar Pradesh-221001, India
Darsh Vithlani	Department of Dyestuff Technology, Institute of Chemical Technology, Mumbai-400019, India
Erik Kellison	Cardiology, CHI Franciscan Heart and Vascular Associates, Tacoma, WA, USA
Guruprasad Mahadevaiah	Cardiology, California North State University College of Medicine, Sacramento, CA, USA
Hatice Feyzan Ay	Yıldız Technical University, Faculty of Chemical and Metallurgical Engineering, Department of Bioengineering, Istanbul, Turkey
Hilal Çalık	Yıldız Technical University, Faculty of Chemical and Metallurgical Engineering, Department of Bioengineering, Istanbul, Turkey
Jyoti Rathee	Department of Chemistry and Center of Advanced Studies in Chemistry, Panjab University, Chandigarh, U.T.-160014, India
Nasir Shariff	Cardiology, CHI Franciscan Heart and Vascular Associates, Tacoma, WA, USA
Neena Mehta	Department of Biochemistry, Rayat Bahra Dental College and Hospital, Mohali, Punjab, India
Prashant Tiwari	School of Pharmacy, Arka Jain University, Jamshedpur, Jharkhand, India
Pratap Kumar Sahu	School of Pharmaceutical Sciences, Siksha O Anusandhan Deemed to be University, Bhuba-neswar, Odisha, 751029, India
Prajakta Dandekar	Department of Pharmaceutical Sciences and Technology, Institute of Chemical Technology, Mumbai-400019, India
Rabia Çakır-Koç	Yıldız Technical University, Faculty of Chemical and Metallurgical Engineering, Department of Bioengineering, Istanbul, Turkey Health Institutes of Turkey (TUSEB), Turkey Biotechnology Institute, Istanbul, Turkey
Rabia Yılmaz	Yıldız Technical University, Faculty of Chemical and Metallurgical Engineering, Department of Bioengineering, Istanbul, Turkey

Ratnesh Jain   Department of Chemical Engineering, Institute of Chemical Technology, Mumbai-400019, India

Rinki Kumari   Department of Microbiology, Hind Institute of Medical Sciences, Mau, Ataria, Sitapur Rd, Uttar Pradesh-261303, India

Rohini Kanwar   Department of Chemistry and Center of Advanced Studies in Chemistry, Panjab University, Chandigarh, U.T.-160014, India

Sathish Chikkabyrappa Cardiology, Seattle Children's Hospital, University of Washington School of Medicine, Seattle,WA, USA

S.K. Mehta   Department of Chemistry and Center of Advanced Studies in Chemistry, Panjab University, Chandigarh, U.T.-160014, India

Snehalata Rai   School of Biomedical Engineering, Indian Institute of Technology (Banaras Hindu University), Varanasi-221005, Uttar Pradesh, India

CHAPTER 1

Effect of Chloroquine and Hydroxychloroquine on the QT Interval in Patients with COVID-19: A Systematic Review

Abdul Aleem[1,*], **Guruprasad Mahadevaiah**[2], **Sathish Chikkabyrappa**[3], **Erik Kellison**[4] and **Nasir Shariff**[4]

[1] *Internal Medicine, Lehigh Valley Hospital, Allentown, PA, USA*

[2] *Cardiology, California North State University College of Medicine, Sacramento, CA, USA*

[3] *Cardiology, Seattle Children's Hospital, University of Washington School of Medicine, Seattle, WA, USA*

[4] *Cardiology, CHI Franciscan Heart and Vascular Associates, Tacoma, WA, USA*

Abstract: Coronavirus disease 2019 (COVID-19) has been a major global health crisis since the influenza pandemic of 1918. Based on data from *in vitro* studies, traditional antimalarial agents, chloroquine and hydroxychloroquine, have been proposed as potential treatment options for patients with COVID-19. Both these medications have also been noted to prolong the QT interval, which increases the risk of drug-induced *torsade de pointes (TdP)* or sudden cardiac death (SCD) when used in non-COVID-19 patients. We reviewed the published clinical studies evaluating the QT interval in COVID-19 patients treated with chloroquine/hydroxychloroquine with or without azithromycin. A literature search using Google Scholar, and PubMed was done for studies published from December 2019 to September 2020. Studies with no specific description of the QT interval were excluded from this review. We identified twelve studies that qualified our criteria, which included 2595 patients. This review addresses the pathophysiology of QT prolongation and the incidence of the magnitude of QT prolongation associated with these medications when used in the treatment of patients admitted with COVID-19. Although most incidences of QT prolongation occurred two or more days after the initiation of these medications, early events of QT prolongation on the first day of therapy have also been reported. Notably, the combination of chloroquine/hydroxychloroquine with azithromycin was associated with a higher incidence of QT prolongation. Although QT prolongation is evident in all the described studies, none of these studies were designed to address the risk of QT prolongation associated with these medications in the outpatient setting or when used as prophylaxis against COVID-19. With the currently available literature, caution with close monitoring of the QT interval is advised when using these antimalarial agents in patients hospitalized with COVID-19 infection.

---

[*] **Corresponding author Abdul Aleem:** Internal Medicine, Lehigh Valley Hospital, Allentown, PA, USA; Tel: 610-402-1415; E-mail: a_aleim@live.com

Keywords: Chloroquine, Coronavirus disease 2019, Covid-19, Drug-induced torsade de pointes (*tdp*), Hydroxychloroquine, Hydroxychloroquine and azithromycin, Qt prolongation, QTc prolongation, SARS-CoV-2, Sudden cardiac death.

INTRODUCTION

COVID-19 caused by a beta coronavirus is included in the same subgenus as the severe acute respiratory syndrome (SARS-CoV) virus. Since the cases of an acute respiratory illness caused by the COVID-19 were initially reported in China in December 2019, the viral infection has spread worldwide, with about four million confirmed cases and more than three hundred thousand death [1]. There has been an urgency to mitigate this illness with experimental therapies and drug repurposing. Currently, there are over 25 potential drugs that are being investigated, with ten in active clinical trials [2]. Traditional antimalarial agents, chloroquine and hydroxychloroquine, have been suggested as potential treatment options for patients with COVID-19 infection based on their *in vitro* activity against the virus [3]. During the early course of the pandemic, the US Food and Drug Administration (FDA) issued an Emergency Use Authorization (EUA), allowing the use of chloroquine and hydroxychloroquine in adult hospitalized patients with COVID-19 outside of a clinical trial . The issuance of the EUA has enabled the conduct of randomized controlled trials(RCTs) to test for the efficacy and safety of these medications [4]. In this systematic review, we aimed to discuss the latest available data regarding the specific complication of QT prolongation associated with the use of chloroquine and hydroxychloroquine in patients with COVID-19 infection.

Pharmacodynamics   and   Pharmacokinetics   of   Chloroquine   and Hydroxychloroquine

Chloroquine is a 9-aminoquinoline that was first synthesized in 1934 from its parent compound quinine, which was derived from the bark of the tropical cinchona tree [5]. Hydroxychloroquine (HCQ) belongs to the same molecular family as chloroquine and differs from its counterpart by the presence of a hydroxyl group [5, 6]. Historically, chloroquine and hydroxychloroquine have been used as antimalarial agents for decades. With the noted immunomodulatory properties of these medications, they have been used widely for the treatment of chronic systemic inflammatory diseases like rheumatoid arthritis and systemic lupus erythematosus [5]. The pharmacokinetics of hydroxychloroquine is similar to that of chloroquine; however, hydroxychloroquine is reported to be less toxic than chloroquine [5]. Both chloroquine and hydroxychloroquine have excellent oral absorption, bioavailability, low blood clearance and, very long half-lives (40 days and 50 days) and are eliminated by hepatic as well as renal excretion [7 - 9].

The antiviral properties of chloroquine have been explored as early as 1987 [10]. *In-vitro* studies have demonstrated the effectiveness of these medications on different RNA viruses, including human immunodeficiency virus (HIV) [6, 11]. However, *in vitro* success of these drugs has not been replicated in clinical trials [6, 12]. *In vitro* studies have shown hydroxychloroquine to inhibit SARS-CoV-2 replication with a 50% maximal effective concentration (EC50) [13]. They are also known to block virus infection by increasing the endosomal pH and interfering with glycosylation of cellular receptors of SARS-CoV [12]. Chloroquine and hydroxychloroquine demonstrate their anti-inflammatory properties by blocking the secretion of pro-inflammatory cytokines such as IFN-gamma, TNF-α, IL-6, and IL-1 [5]. This anti-inflammatory action of chloroquine and hydroxychloroquine has been hypothesized to be beneficial in countering the inappropriate immune activation by SARS-CoV-2, leading to ARDS [14].

Effect of Chloroquine and Hydroxychloroquine Against SARS-CoV-2

In vitro Studies

Based on previous preclinical data demonstrating hydroxychloroquine having anti-SARS-CoV activity in the last SARS outbreak [15], Yao *et al.* studied the activity of chloroquine and hydroxychloroquine *in vitro* against SARS-CoV-2. Hydroxychloroquine was noted to be more effective than chloroquine *in vitro* against SARS-CoV-2 infection [3]. Liu *et al.* also described the positive effect of chloroquine and hydroxychloroquine on SARS-CoV-2 *in vitro* and concluded hydroxychloroquine to be superior to chloroquine in inhibiting SARS-CoV-2 *in vitro*. Chloroquine was associated with a significant reduction in quantitative real-time ET-PCR viral load in Vero E6 cells infected with SARS-CoV [13]. Chloroquine was also noted to inhibit the entry and post-entry stages of the SARS-CoV virus at fluid concentrations, which could be achieved at doses usually used in patients with rheumatoid arthritis [9, 16].

In vivo Studies

Data from several initial nonrandomized control studies showed significant improvement in clinical symptoms and early viral conversion rates with the use of hydroxychloroquine and chloroquine in patients with COVID-19 [17 - 20]. These studies, however, did not address the cardiac adverse effects of these medications, precisely their effect on QT interval by these medications. Data from further observational studies examining the clinical efficacy of these drugs could not replicate the positive results demonstrated by the initial trials [21 - 23]. A double-masked randomized control trial by Borba *et al.* in Brazil involving 81 severely ill patients who were randomized to receive a high and low dosage of chloroquine, which was given concurrently with azithromycin and oseltamivir, was abruptly halted due to the high mortality rate noted during the study which was 39% in the top dosage group and 15% in the low dosage group, respectively [24]. There was an observed association of the use of these medications with QT prolongation and poor outcomes [23, 24].

Effect on the QT Interval

Ventricular repolarization duration and the QT interval are determined by the ventricular action potential [25]. In contrast to the QRS duration, the QT interval varies with heart rate and autonomic tone. The outward potassium currents occur due to the two delayed rectifying channels, - *IKr* (rapid) and *IKs* (slow) channels. The inhibition or reduction of the *IKr* channel activity is the primary cause of prolongation of the QT interval. Secondary to the reduced *IKr* channel activity, some L-type calcium channels (which are inactive during depolarization) may become activated, resulting in early afterdepolarization, which in turn results in triggered arrhythmia facilitating polymorphic ventricular tachycardia. Any change or defect in the function of ion channels and related proteins of the ventricular myocytes leads to abnormal repolarization of the ventricular myocardium, which results in the prolongation of the QT interval on the electrocardiogram (ECG) [26]. These defects can be congenital, drug-induced, or due to electrolyte abnormalities. Several medications that include macrolides, fluoroquinolones, antipsychotics, and antiarrhythmic drugs that block potassium channels are known to prolong the QT interval. Amongst the different classes of antimalarial medications, quinolines, and structurally related antimalarial drugs like chloroquine and hydroxychloroquine have clinically substantial cardiovascular effects [27]. Chloroquine and hydroxychloroquine are known to cause prolongation of QT interval by inhibiting the rapidly activating delayed rectifier K+ current (*IKr*) encoded by a cardiac potassium channel gene called the human-*ether-a-go-go-related gene* (hERG). This blockade causes a decrease in the net repolarizing current leading to an increase in the duration of ventricular action potential manifesting as a prolonged QT interval, which can potentially cause life-threatening ventricular arrhythmias like torsades de pointes or sudden cardiac death (SCD) [26, 28, 29].

Effect on the QT Interval in Patients with COVID-19

Chloroquine and hydroxychloroquine have been demonstrated to cause prolongation of the QT interval when used to manage patients with malaria and rheumatoid arthritis [30]. There are also several case reports of polymorphic ventricular tachycardia in non-COVID-19 patients receiving these medications [31, 32]. The first randomized control trial (Table **1**) evaluating the clinical efficacy and safety of chloroquine in patients with severe COVID-19 was published by Borba *et al.* [24]. In this prospective study evaluating the safety and clinical efficacy chloroquine, 81 patients with severe COVID-19 illness were randomized into two groups to receive either high dosage chloroquine (600mg twice daily for ten days) or low dosage chloroquine (450mg twice a day for the first day followed by once a day for four days). All patients received ceftriaxone and azithromycin as well. There were significantly higher events of QT prolongation in the higher dose group compared to the lower dose group (18.9% *vs.* 11.1%). Two patients in the high dosage arm developed ventricular tachycardia prior to their death. The study was terminated early due to its high mortality rate in the high dosage group compared to the low dosage group [24].

Table 1. Summary of the published prospective/retrospective studies describing the effect of chloroquine and/or hydroxychloroquine in combination with or without azithromycin on QT interval in patients hospitalized with COVID-19 illness.

Author	Study Design	Objective	Sample Size(N)	Baseline QTc Interval(ms)	Effect on QT Interval	Results
Borba *et al.* [24]	Double masked randomized control trial	Evaluate the safety and efficacy of high dosage chloroquine (600mg twice daily for 10 days) and low dosage chloroquine (450mg twice a day for the first day followed by once a day for 4 days) in hospitalized patients with severe COVID-19 infection	N=81 High dosage group:40 Low dosage group:41	**High dosage group**: 421.9 ± 24.0 **Low dosage group**: 427.8 ± 31.0	QTc interval (>500 ms) noted in 7 patients (18.9%) in the high dosage group compared with 4 patients (11.1%) in the low-dosage group	Study was terminated due to trends towards a higher lethality rate of 39% in the high dosage group and 15% in the low dosage group. Ventricular arrhythmia developed in 2/37 patients of the high dose chloroquine arm and 0/28 in the low dose arm

(Table 1) contd.....

Author	Study Design	Objective	Sample Size(N)	Baseline QTc Interval(ms)	Effect on QT Interval	Results
Rosenberg *et al.* [22]	Retrospective multicenter cohort study	Evaluate mortality in hospitalized patients receiving HCQ, AZ, both or neither	**N=1438** **HCQ plus AZ:** (735) **HCQ alone**: (271) **AZ alone:** (211) **Neither drug:** (221)	Not specified	**HCQ plus AZ:**12.6% (80 patients) **HCQ alone**:16.7% (39 patients) **AZ alone**:8.3% (15 patients) Neither drug:8.4%	Compared to patients receiving neither HCQ or AZ, higher mortality was noted in patients receiving these medications: HCQ alone (HR, 1.08) combination HCQ with AZ (HR, 1.35) AZ alone (HR, 0.56) Adjusted cardiac arrest events were significantly higher in patients receiving a combination of AZ and HCQ when compared to patients receiving neither of the medications (HR 2.97)

(Table 1) contd.....

Author	Study Design	Objective	Sample Size(N)	Baseline QTc Interval(ms)	Effect on QT Interval	Results
Mercuro *et al.* [33]	Retrospective single center study	Assess the QT prolongation in patients receiving HCQ with or without concomitant AZ	**N=90** **Concomitant AZ with HCQ:** (53) **HCQ alone:** (37)	**Overall**:455 (430-474) ms **HCQ**: 473 (454-487) ms **HCQ and AZ**: 442 (427-461) ms	10 of 90 patients (11%) had ΔQTc of 60 ms or more; 18 (20%) had post treatment QTc intervals of 500 ms or more. **HCQ monotherapy**: 7 (19%) developed QTc > 500 ms and 3 (3%) had ΔQTc > 60 ms **Concomitant AZ**: 11 (21%) had QTc > 500ms and 7 (13%) had a ΔQTc > 60 ms	High risk of QT prolongation was noted in patients receiving HCQ 1 patient on HCQ developed Torsades de Pointes
Bessière *et al.* [34]	Prospective single center case series study	Examine the effect and safety of HCQ with or without AZ on QT interval in ICU patients	**N=40** **HCQ alone:** (22) **In association with AZ:** (18)	414 (392-428) ms	93% of the patients showed an increase in QTc after receiving HCQ with or without AZ. QTc > 500ms in 6 patients (33%) receiving HCQ with AZ and 1 patient (5%) receiving HCQ alone 10 patients with Δ QTc >60 ms Total patients with prolonged QTc -14	High incidence of QT prolongation in patients receiving HCQ

(Table 1) contd.....

Author	Study Design	Objective	Sample Size(N)	Baseline QTc Interval(ms)	Effect on QT Interval	Results
Saleh *et al.* [35]	Prospective observational study	Examine the effect of Chloroquine, HCQ and AZ on the QTc interval in hospitalized patients with COVID-19	**Monotherapy group:**201 chloroquine (10) HCQ: 191) **Combination group:** (chloroquine/HCQ and AZ):119	**Monotherapy group:** 440.6 ± 24.9 **Combination group:** 439.9 ± 24.7	Maximum QTc was significantly longer in the combination group 470.4 ± 45.0 ms *vs.* 453.3 ± 37.0 in the monotherapy group **QTC >500 ms:** 7 patients in monotherapy *vs.* 11 patients in combination therapy	No instances of TdP or arrhythmogenic death QT prolongation was noted after day 1 of treatment 7 patients (2 on monotherapy) required discontinuation of these medications due to QTc prolongation 7 Patients-non sustained monomorphic ventricular tachycardia 1 patient had sustained monomorphic tachycardia in the setting of viral myocarditis 17 patients developed new onset atrial fibrillation

(Table 1) contd.....

Author	Study Design	Objective	Sample Size(N)	Baseline QTc Interval(ms)	Effect on QT Interval	Results
Chorin *et al.* [36]	Retrospective multicenter study	Assess the progression of QTc and incidence of arrhythmia and mortality in patients treated with HCQ/AZ	N=251	QTc:439 ±29 ms (QT interval assessed at baseline and up to 3 days of completion of therapy)	58 /251 (23%) patients treated with HCQ/AZ developed extreme new QTc prolongation of > 500 ms. The QTc interval prolonged from 439 ± 29 ms at baseline to 473 ± 36 ms ($P < .001$) with therapy.	The combination of HCQ/AZ significantly prolonged the QTc predisposing to life threatening arrhythmia Maximum QT prolongation was noted 4 ± 2 days of therapy. One patient developed **polymorphic ventricular tachycardia** requiring defibrillation
Ramireddy *et al.* [37]	Retrospective single center study	Examine the effect of HCQ, AZ or both on the QTc Interval	**N=98 AZ**:27 **HCQ**:10 **Combination (AZ/HCQ):** 61	448±29 ms	Overall QTc increased to 459±36ms ($p=0.005$) with drug administration with the highest mean change in QTc values in the combined HCQ and AZ group 12% of patients reached critical QTc prolongation	QTc prolongation was several folds higher with combination therapy compared to AZ alone (17±39 ms *versus* 0.5±40 ms; $p=0.07$).

Author	Study Design	Objective	Sample Size(N)	Baseline QTc Interval(ms)	Effect on QT Interval	Results
Mahevas *et al.* [38]	Retrospective cohort study	Assess effectiveness of HCQ in admitted patients on oxygen (non-ICU)	N=181 **HCQ:** (84) **Control:** 89	Not specified	7/84 had QTc increase > 60 ms, of which one had QTc> 500 ms	At day 21, overall survival was 89% in treated *vs.* 91% in the control group Rate of survival was 69% in treated *vs.* 74% in control on day 21
Perinel *et al* [39]	Prospective single center cohort study	Evaluate the pharmacokinetic properties of HCQ (200 mg TID PO) in ICU COVID 19 patients	N=13	Not specified	Dosage of HCQ needed to be reduced in 4 patients (200 mg of HCQ twice daily) due to increased levels of HCQ on blood samples. Two patients needed withdrawal of the medication due to QT interval prolongation (381 to 510 ms and 432 to 550 ms) on day 2 and 3, respectively	Only 8/13 patients achieved the minimum therapeutic level of 1 mg/ml. QT prolongation noted on day 2 and day 3 of treatment in 2/13 patients
Molina *et al.* [40]	Prospective single center study	Study the virologic and clinical outcomes of treatment with HCQ and AZ	N=11	Not specified	One patient was noted to have QT interval prolongation from 405 ms to 460 and 470 ms requiring discontinuation of therapy	Repeat nasopharyngeal swabs were positive in 8 of the 10 patients at 5 days

(Table 1) contd.....

Author	Study Design	Objective	Sample Size(N)	Baseline QTc Interval(ms)	Effect on QT Interval	Results
Voisin *et al.* [41]	Prospective single center study	Examine the effect of HCQ and AZ on the QTc Interval by analysing serial ECGs recorded in patients hospitalized with COVID-19 pneumonia and treated with both HCQ and AZ	N=50	QTc:408 ms at baseline (IQR, 343-478 ms) (QT interval assessed at base and at day 3, at day 5 and at discharge)	Mean QTc interval increased up to 437 ms (IQR, 380-500 ms) at day 3 and to 456 ms (IQR, 397-518 ms) at day 5 Median QTc interval at day 0, day 3, and day 5 was 403, 430, and 460 ms, respectively 38 patients (76%) had short-term modifications of the QTc duration (>30 ms) 6 patients (12%) had treatment discontinuation	The combination of HCQ and AZ used in short duration significantly prolong the QTc interval necessitating cardiac monitoring at regular intervals
Cipriani *et al.* [42]	Prospective single center study	Examine the effect of HCQ and AZ on the QTc interval with 12 lead 24-hour Holter monitoring in patients hospitalized with COVID-19 pneumonia	N=22	QTc:426 ms at baseline (IQR, 403-447 ms)	QTc interval increased up to 450 ms (IQR, 416-476 ms) 4 patients had QTc ≥ 480ms	Therapy with HCQ and AZ prolongs the QTc interval. Multiple daily ECG is not recommended due to stability in the QTc duration

Abbreviations: QTc, corrected QT; HCQ, Hydroxychloroquine; ms, milliseconds; AZ, Azithromycin; TdP, torsades de Pointes; ΔQTc, change in corrected QT interval; IQR, Interquartile range; ECG, Electro-cardiogram;

In a large retrospective multicenter observational cohort study of 1438 patients admitted with COVID-19, the adjusted hazard ratio for in-hospital mortality for treatment with hydroxychloroquine alone was 1.08 and when combined with azithromycin was 1.35 when compared to patients receiving neither of these medications. The combination of azithromycin with hydroxychloroquine was associated with higher events of cardiac arrests as compared to patients receiving neither of these medications (15.5% *vs.* 6.8%). QTc prolongation was noted in 12.6% receiving azithromycin with hydroxychloroquine, 16.7% in patients receiving hydroxychloroquine, and 8.4% receiving neither of the medications [22].

Mercuro *et al.* reported a change in QT interval in a cohort of 90 hospitalized patients who had received hydroxychloroquine with or without azithromycin [33]. The median baseline QTc was 455 (430-474) msec. Patients receiving the combination of hydroxychloroquine and azithromycin had a more considerable increase in QT interval (23 {10-40} msec) compared with those receiving hydroxychloroquine alone (5.5 {−15.5 to 34.25} [1] msec) (p=0.03) Of the 53 receiving combined therapy, 11 (13%) had prolonged QTc over 500 msec, and 7 (13%) had a change in QTc of 60 msec or more. One patient on combination therapy developed QT prolongation (499 msec) and torsades de pointes three days later. In a single-center French study of 40 patients admitted to intensive care unit receiving hydroxychloroquine (200mg twice a day for ten days) of which 45% of patients also received azithromycin reported that 93% of patients showed an increase in QTc with seven patients (18%) having QTc interval over 500msec [34]. The prolongation of the QT interval was noted after 3 to 5 days of being on therapy.

Another prospective observational study examined the effect of chloroquine, hydroxychloroquine, and azithromycin on QTc interval in 201 patients hospitalized with COVID-19, in which ten patients received chloroquine while 191 patients received hydroxychloroquine [35]. In patients receiving a combination of hydroxychloroquine/chloroquine with azithromycin, the QT prolongation was significantly longer than patients receiving hydroxychloroquine/chloroquine without azithromycin (470±45 msec *versus* 453 ±37 msec, P=0.004). Seven patients (3.5%) required discontinuation of the medications due to the significant prolongation of the QT intervals. There were no reported instances of *TdP* or arrhythmogenic death in patients receiving either drug or in combination. However, seven patients experienced non-sustained monomorphic tachycardia and one patient with sustained monomorphic tachycardia in the setting of viral myocarditis. There was also new-onset atrial fibrillation reported in 17 patients.

Electrocardiographic measures at baseline and up to 3 days of completion of therapy in 251 patients who received hydroxychloroquine with azithromycin noted prolongation of the QT interval in patients receiving these medications with incomplete resolution of the QT interval after completion of the therapy [36]. About 23% of patients developed extreme QT prolongation of over 500msec, and one patient developed polymorphic ventricular tachycardia requiring defibrillation. QTc prolongation was noted from 439 ± 29 msec at baseline to 473 ± 36 msec (P < .001) with therapy. Maximum QT prolongation was observed to be 4.1 ± 2 days of being on therapy [36].

In a case series of 98 patients with COVID-19 treated with azithromycin (28%), hydroxychloroquine (10%), or a combination (62%) of both medications, baseline QTc interval was 448±29 msec and increased to 459±36 msec (p=0.005) with the administration of these drugs [37]. 12% of patients reached critical QTc prolongation with the combination therapy group, demonstrating the highest QTc prolongation. Combination therapy had a significant increase in QTc prolongation when compared with azithromycin therapy (17±39 msec *versus* 0.5±40 msec; p=0.07). None of the patients developed polymorphic ventricular tachycardia.

Mahevas *et al.* reported a study of 181 patients receiving non-intensive care (on oxygen therapy) due to COVID-19 pneumonia, of which 84 patients received hydroxychloroquine (600mg/day) [38]. Among the patients receiving hydroxychloroquine, the overall survival rate was 89% at 21 days compared to 91% in the control group (HR 1.2, 0.4 to 3.3). Of the 84 patients who received hydroxychloroquine, eight (10%) experienced EKG changes requiring discontinuation of hydroxychloroquine at a median interval of 4 days (interquartile range 3-9 days). Seven patients had a QTc interval prolongation of more than 60 msec, and one patient had QTc of more than 500 msec.

Thirteen patients with COVID-19 admitted to the intensive care unit received hydroxychloroquine 200 mg three times a day in a prospective study of which twelve patients received ventilator support while one patient received extracorporeal membrane oxygenation (ECMO) [39]. The dosage of hydroxychloroquine needed to be reduced in 4 patients (200 mg of hydroxychloroquine twice daily) due to higher levels of hydroxychloroquine on blood samples, while two patients required withdrawal of the medication due to QT interval prolongation (381 to 510 ms and 432 to 550 msec) on day 2 and 3. In a small prospective study involving 11 hospitalized patients, virologic and clinical outcomes with therapy with hydroxychloroquine (600 mg/d for ten days) and azithromycin (500 mg day 1 and 250 mg days 2 to 5) were evaluated [40]. 80% of patients had persistent positive virology studies despite therapy of over five days. One patient developed a significant prolongation of the QT interval from 405 to 470, which required discontinuation of the therapy on day 4. ECG analysis of 50 patients treated with hydroxychloroquine and azithromycin at baseline, day 3 and day 5 of treatment in a single center prospective study reported increase in QT interval in 76% patients with treatment discontinuation in 12% of patients [41].QT interval was noted to be prolonged in another prospective single center study that examined the role of 24 hour Holter monitoring of patients treated with hydroxychloroquine and azithromycin. However, this study recommended checking daily serial ECGs due to 24-hour stability in the QT interval in patients receiving these drugs [42].

Consistent with each of these described studies, the use of these medications has been employed in only hospitalized patients with COVID-19. A substantial proportion of patients also received azithromycin, which has also been implicated in prolonging the QT interval. Currently, there have been no studies addressing the QT interval with the use of using these drugs in the outpatient setting. There has been no documented evidence of the occurrence of polymorphic ventricular tachycardia when using hydroxychloroquine or chloroquine as prophylactic agents to prevent COVID- 19 infection. Further studies are required to address these specific situations and in defining the role of the use of these medications in COVID-19.

CONCLUSION

Although *in-vitro* studies have shown the inhibition of the SARS-CoV virus by the conventional antimalarial agents' chloroquine and hydroxychloroquine, there has been a significant concern of QT prolongation when used as a treatment in patients hospitalized with COVID-19 infection. The concurrent use of azithromycin with these agents has been noted to have an additive effect on prolongation of the QT interval. Most events of QT prolongation occurred two days after the initiation of the therapy; however, QT prolongation has also been reported to occur after day 1 of treatment. All the published studies were in admitted patients with COVID- 19 infection. There has been no study to address the role of these medications when used to treat patients with a less severe infection in the outpatient setting or when used as a prophylactic agent. With the available literature, it is prudent to closely monitor QT interval prolongation and drug-drug interactions when using these antimalarial medications to treat hospitalized patients with COVID-19 infection.

CONSENT FOR PUBLICATION

Not applicable.

CONFLICT OF INTEREST

The author declares no conflict of interest, financial or otherwise.

ACKNOWLEDGEMENTS

Declared none.

REFERENCES

[1]   World Health Organization. 2020. Available from: https://www.who.int/dg/speeches/detail/who-director-general-s-opening-remarks-at-the-media-briefing-on-covid-19---11-march-2020

[2]   Rome BN, Avorn J. Drug evaluation during the Covid-19 pandemic. N Engl J Med 2020; 382(24): 2282-4.
[http://dx.doi.org/10.1056/NEJMp2009457] [PMID: 32289216]

[3]   Yao X, Ye F, Zhang M, *et al. In Vitro* Antiviral Activity and Projection of Optimized Dosing Design of Hydroxychloroquine for the Treatment of Severe Acute Respiratory Syndrome Coronavirus 2 (SARS-CoV-2). Clin Infect Dis 2020; 71(15): 732-9.
[http://dx.doi.org/10.1093/cid/ciaa237] [PMID: 32150618]

[4]   Gandhi RT, Lynch JB, Del Rio C. Mild or moderate COVID-19. N Engl J Med 2020; 383(18): 1757-66.
[http://dx.doi.org/10.1056/NEJMcp2009249] [PMID: 32329974]

[5]   Savarino A, Boelaert JR, Cassone A, Majori G, Cauda R. Effects of chloroquine on viral infections: an old drug against today's diseases? Lancet Infect Dis 2003; 3(11): 722-7.
[http://dx.doi.org/10.1016/S1473-3099(03)00806-5] [PMID: 14592603]

[6]   Devaux CA, Rolain J-M, Colson P, Raoult D. New insights on the antiviral effects of chloroquine against coronavirus: what to expect for COVID-19? Int J Antimicrob Agents 2020; 55(5): 105938.
[http://dx.doi.org/10.1016/j.ijantimicag.2020.105938] [PMID: 32171740]

[7]   Stokkermans TJ, Trichonas G. New insights on the antiviral effects of chloroquine against coronavirus: what to expect for COVID-19? Int J Antimicrob Agents 2020; 105938.

[8]   Furst DE. Pharmacokinetics of hydroxychloroquine and chloroquine during treatment of rheumatic diseases. Lupus 1996; 5(1_suppl): 11-5.
[http://dx.doi.org/10.1177/0961203396005001041]

[9]   Mackenzie AH. Pharmacologic actions of 4-aminoquinoline compounds. Am J Med 1983; 75(1A): 5-10.
[http://dx.doi.org/10.1016/0002-9343(83)91264-0] [PMID: 6603166]

[10]   Krogstad DJ, Schlesinger PH. Acid-vesicle function, intracellular pathogens, and the action of chloroquine against Plasmodium falciparum. N Engl J Med 1987; 317(9): 542-9.
[http://dx.doi.org/10.1056/NEJM198708273170905] [PMID: 3302712]

[11]   Boelaert JR, Piette J, Sperber K. The potential place of chloroquine in the treatment of HIV-1-infected patients. J Clin Virol 2001; 20(3): 137-40.
[http://dx.doi.org/10.1016/S1386-6532(00)00140-2] [PMID: 11166662]

[12]   Vincent MJ, Bergeron E, Benjannet S, *et al.* Chloroquine is a potent inhibitor of SARS coronavirus infection and spread. Virol J 2005; 2(1): 69.
[http://dx.doi.org/10.1186/1743-422X-2-69] [PMID: 16115318]

[13]   Liu J, Cao R, Xu M, *et al.* Hydroxychloroquine, a less toxic derivative of chloroquine, is effective in inhibiting SARS-CoV-2 infection *in vitro.* Cell Discov 2020; 6(1): 16.
[http://dx.doi.org/10.1038/s41421-020-0156-0] [PMID: 32194981]

[14]   Zhou D, Dai S-M, Tong Q. COVID-19: a recommendation to examine the effect of hydroxychloroquine in preventing infection and progression. J Antimicrob Chemother 2020; 75(7): 1667-70.
[http://dx.doi.org/10.1093/jac/dkaa114] [PMID: 32196083]

[15]   Savarino A, Di Trani L, Donatelli I, Cauda R, Cassone A. New insights into the antiviral effects of chloroquine. Lancet Infect Dis 2006; 6(2): 67-9.
[http://dx.doi.org/10.1016/S1473-3099(06)70361-9] [PMID: 16439323]

[16]   Wang M, Cao R, Zhang L, *et al.* Remdesivir and chloroquine effectively inhibit the recently emerged

novel coronavirus (2019-nCoV) *in vitro.* Cell Res 2020; 30(3): 269-71.
[http://dx.doi.org/10.1038/s41422-020-0282-0] [PMID: 32020029]

[17] Gao J, Tian Z, Yang X. Breakthrough: Chloroquine phosphate has shown apparent efficacy in treatment of COVID-19 associated pneumonia in clinical studies. Biosci Trends 2020; 14(1): 72-3.
[http://dx.doi.org/10.5582/bst.2020.01047] [PMID: 32074550]

[18] Chen J, Liu D, Liu L, *et al.* A pilot study of hydroxychloroquine in treatment of patients with moderate COVID-19. Zhejiang da xue xue bao Yi xue ban= Journal of Zhejiang University Medical sciences 2020; 49(2).

[19] Chen Z, Hu J, Zhang Z, *et al.* Efficacy of hydroxychloroquine in patients with COVID-19: results of a randomized clinical trial. MedRxiv 2020.

[20] Gautret P, Lagier J-C, Parola P, *et al.* Hydroxychloroquine and azithromycin as a treatment of COVID-19: results of an open-label non-randomized clinical trial. Int J Antimicrob Agents 2020; 56(1): 105949.
[http://dx.doi.org/10.1016/j.ijantimicag.2020.105949] [PMID: 32205204]

[21] Geleris J, Sun Y, Platt J, *et al.* Observational study of hydroxychloroquine in hospitalized patients with Covid-19. N Engl J Med 2020; 382(25): 2411-8.
[http://dx.doi.org/10.1056/NEJMoa2012410] [PMID: 32379955]

[22] Rosenberg ES, Dufort EM, Udo T, *et al.* Association of treatment with hydroxychloroquine or azithromycin with in-hospital mortality in patients with COVID-19 in New York state. JAMA 2020; 323(24): 2493-502.
[http://dx.doi.org/10.1001/jama.2020.8630] [PMID: 32392282]

[23] Magagnoli J, Narendran S, Pereira F, *et al.* Outcomes of hydroxychloroquine usage in United States veterans hospitalized with Covid-19. Med 2020.

[24] Borba MGS, Val FFA, Sampaio VS, *et al.* Effect of high *vs.* low doses of chloroquine diphosphate as adjunctive therapy for patients hospitalized with severe acute respiratory syndrome coronavirus 2 (SARS-CoV-2) infection: a randomized clinical trial. JAMA network open 2020; 3(4): e208857.

[25] Roden D. The long QT syndrome and torsades de pointes: basic and clinical aspects Cardiac pacing and electrophysiology. Philadelphia: WB Saunders 1991; pp. 265-83.

[26] Drew BJ, Ackerman MJ, Funk M, *et al.* American Heart Association Acute Cardiac Care Committee of the Council on Clinical Cardiology, the Council on Cardiovascular Nursing, and the American College of Cardiology Foundation. Prevention of torsade de pointes in hospital settings: a scientific statement from the American Heart Association and the American College of Cardiology Foundation. Circulation 2010; 121(8): 1047-60.
[http://dx.doi.org/10.1161/CIRCULATIONAHA.109.192704] [PMID: 20142454]

[27] White NJ. Cardiotoxicity of antimalarial drugs. Lancet Infect Dis 2007; 7(8): 549-58.
[http://dx.doi.org/10.1016/S1473-3099(07)70187-1] [PMID: 17646028]

[28] Traebert M, Dumotier B, Meister L, Hoffmann P, Dominguez-Estevez M, Suter W. Inhibition of hERG K+ currents by antimalarial drugs in stably transfected HEK293 cells. Eur J Pharmacol 2004; 484(1): 41-8.
[http://dx.doi.org/10.1016/j.ejphar.2003.11.003] [PMID: 14729380]

[29] Capel RA, Herring N, Kalla M, *et al.* Hydroxychloroquine reduces heart rate by modulating the hyperpolarization-activated current If: Novel electrophysiological insights and therapeutic potential. Heart Rhythm 2015; 12(10): 2186-94.
[http://dx.doi.org/10.1016/j.hrthm.2015.05.027] [PMID: 26025323]

[30] Ursing J, Rombo L, Eksborg S, *et al.* High-dose chloroquine for uncomplicated plasmodium falciparum malaria is well tolerated and causes similar QT interval prolongation as standard-dose chloroquine in children. Antimicrob Agents Chemother 2020; 64(3): e01846-19.
[http://dx.doi.org/10.1128/AAC.01846-19] [PMID: 31907183]

[31] O'Laughlin JP, Mehta PH, Wong BC. Life threatening severe QTc prolongation in patient with systemic lupus erythematosus due to hydroxychloroquine. Case reports in cardiology 2016; 2016
[http://dx.doi.org/10.1155/2016/4626279]

[32] Wroblewski HA, Kovacs RJ, Kingery JR, Overholser BR, Tisdale JE. High risk of QT interval prolongation and torsades de pointes associated with intravenous quinidine used for treatment of resistant malaria or babesiosis. Antimicrob Agents Chemother 2012; 56(8): 4495-9.
[http://dx.doi.org/10.1128/AAC.06396-11] [PMID: 22615288]

[33] Mercuro NJ, Yen CF, Shim DJ, *et al.* Risk of QT interval prolongation associated with use of hydroxychloroquine with or without concomitant azithromycin among hospitalized patients testing positive for coronavirus disease 2019 (COVID-19). JAMA Cardiol 2020; 5(9): 1036-41.
[http://dx.doi.org/10.1001/jamacardio.2020.1834] [PMID: 32936252]

[34] Bessière F, Roccia H, Delinière A, *et al.* Assessment of QT Intervals in a case series of patients with coronavirus disease 2019 (COVID-19) infection treated with hydroxychloroquine alone or in combination with azithromycin in an intensive care unit. JAMA Cardiol 2020; 5(9): 1067-9.
[http://dx.doi.org/10.1001/jamacardio.2020.1787] [PMID: 32936266]

[35] Saleh M, Gabriels J, Chang D, *et al.* The effect of chloroquine, hydroxychloroquine and azithromycin on the corrected QT interval in patients with SARS-CoV-2 infection. Circ Arrhythm Electrophysiol 2020; 13(6): e008662.
[http://dx.doi.org/10.1161/CIRCEP.120.008662] [PMID: 32347743]

[36] Chorin E, Wadhwani L, Magnani S, *et al.* QT interval prolongation and torsade de pointes in patients with COVID-19 treated with hydroxychloroquine/azithromycin. Heart Rhythm 2020; 17(9): 1425-33.
[http://dx.doi.org/10.1016/j.hrthm.2020.05.014] [PMID: 32407884]

[37] Ramireddy A, Chugh H, Reinier K, *et al.* Experience With Hydroxychloroquine and Azithromycin in the Coronavirus Disease 2019 Pandemic: Implications for QT Interval Monitoring. J Am Heart Assoc 2020; 9(12): e017144.
[http://dx.doi.org/10.1161/JAHA.120.017144] [PMID: 32463348]

[38] Mahevas M, Tran V-T, Roumier M, *et al.* No evidence of clinical efficacy of hydroxychloroquine in patients hospitalized for COVID-19 infection with oxygen requirement: results of a study using routinely collected data to emulate a target trial. MedRxiv 2020.

[39] Perinel S, Launay M, Botelho-Nevers É, *et al.* Towards optimization of hydroxychloroquine dosing in intensive care unit COVID-19 patients. Clin Infect Dis 2020; 71(16): 2227-9.
[http://dx.doi.org/10.1093/cid/ciaa394] [PMID: 32255489]

[40] Molina JM, Delaugerre C, Le Goff J, *et al.* No evidence of rapid antiviral clearance or clinical benefit with the combination of hydroxychloroquine and azithromycin in patients with severe COVID-19 infection. Med Mal Infect 2020; 50(4): 384.
[http://dx.doi.org/10.1016/j.medmal.2020.03.006] [PMID: 32240719]

[41] Voisin O, Lorc'h EL, Mahé A, *et al.* Acute QT Interval Modifications During Hydroxychloroquine-Azithromycin Treatment in the Context of COVID-19 Infection. Mayo Clin Proc 2020; 95(8): 1696-700.
[http://dx.doi.org/10.1016/j.mayocp.2020.05.005] [PMID: 32753141]

[42] Cipriani A, Zorzi A, Ceccato D, *et al.* Arrhythmic profile and 24-hour QT interval variability in COVID-19 patients treated with hydroxychloroquine and azithromycin. Int J Cardiol 2020; 316: 280-4.
[http://dx.doi.org/10.1016/j.ijcard.2020.05.036] [PMID: 32439366]

CHAPTER 2

COVID-19: Impact of Pandemic on SAARC Nations

Rohini Kanwar[1], Jyoti Rathee[1], Amit Kumar[1], Neena Mehta[2] and S. K. Mehta[1,*]

[1] *Department of Chemistry and Center of Advanced Studies in Chemistry, Panjab University, Chandigarh, U.T.-160014, India*

[2] *Department of Biochemistry, Rayat Bahra Dental College and Hospital, Mohali, Punjab, India*

Abstract: The recent outbreak of Severe Acute Respiratory Syndrome CoronaVirus 2 (SARS-CoV-2), from Wuhan, China, has turned out to be a global pandemic after sustained human to human transmission. While developed nations like the USA, Spain, Italy, Germany, and so forth have not been able to handle the episode, the situation at the moment is devastating in the South Asian Association for Regional Cooperation Countries, popularly known as SAARC countries. The present report is an attempt to understand the measurable correlation of the coronavirus cases, casualties, and mortality rates in the SAARC nations. It also analyses the drugs being tested in these countries to battle against the deadly virus. Moreover, the response of SAARC nations against COVID-19 and the effect of lockdown on daily life, economy, environment, and education have been discussed. Finally, to mitigate the COVID-19 pandemic, a strategy has been chalked down based on the knowledge obtained from the rest of the world.

Keywords: COVID-19, Coronavirus, COVID pandemic, Economy, Environment, Mortality rate, Mitigation, Pandemic 2020, SARS-CoV-2, SAARC nations.

INTRODUCTION

An outbreak of a Severe Acute Respiratory Syndrome CoronaVirus disease 2019 (COVID-19) from Wuhan, China, has been declared a global pandemic by the World Health Organization (WHO) on 11th March 2020. SARS-CoV-2 is a beta Coronavirus like MERS-CoV and SARS-CoV. A group of researchers believes that coronavirus may have spread from animals (bats) to humans *via* pangolin and later spread through human - to - human contact, which afterward led to an

---

* **Corresponding author S. K. Mehta :** Department of Chemistry and Center of Advanced Studies in Chemistry, Panjab University, Chandigarh, U.T.-160014, India; E-mail: skmehta@pu.ac.in

Jean-Marc Sabatier (Ed.)

international community spread. The structure of SARS-CoV-2 has been shown in Fig. (**1**) [1]. The whole world has come under the effect of this Chinese originated virus, where a total count of positive cases has gone to 50,250,314, and deaths have risen to 1,255,906 (by 6th November 2020). (Source: Worldometer)

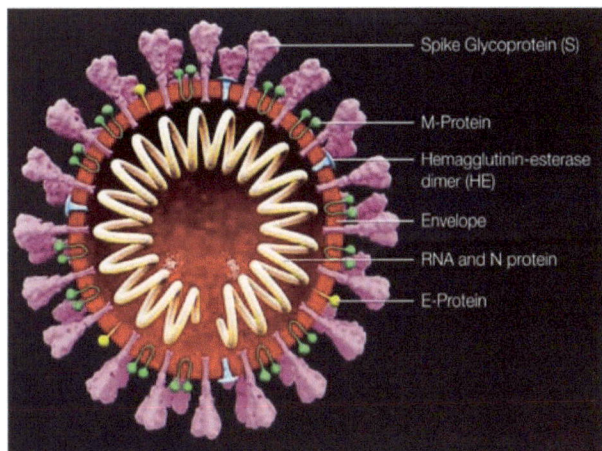

Fig. (1).   Structure of SARS-CoV-2 https://www.scientificanimations.com/coronavirus-symptoms-a-d-prevention-explained-through-medical-animation/.

China is a growing economic player that has always tried to play a strategic role in neighboring countries. Despite being only an observer in the South Asian Association for Regional Cooperation (SAARC), its role has been the most discussed one and has always been seeking an expansion. With an outbreak of this deadly virus, China has greatly impacted the SAARC nations. Although this SARS-CoV-2 virus has drastically affected the whole world, it is important to visualize the impact of this deadly virus on economically struck developing nations grouping referred to as SAARC. Since the impact of this virus on the European nations has been constantly documented, no such report has been written on SAARC nations. Moreover, SAARC countries make up 21% of the total world population, so the fate of the world post-COVID-19 will be largely dependent on COVID-19 impact on SAARC nations.

The SAARC is the regional intergovernmental organization and geopolitical union of states in South Asia. It is a cluster of 8 countries, namely, Afghanistan, Bangladesh, Bhutan, India, the Maldives, Nepal, Pakistan, and Sri Lanka. It was established on 8th December 1985 in Dhaka. Its dialogue is often conducted in the form of SAARC meetings to promote economic and regional integration. In this pandemic time, to chart out a common strategy to combat the COVID-19 in the region, India initiated a SAARC video conference on 15th March 2020. India offered the establishment of a rapid response team of doctors and specialists, online training capsules, sharing of software, common research platform, evacuation of citizens, *etc.*, as relief measures during the video conference. As a way forward, the COVID-19 Emergency fund was proposed on voluntary contributions from all the countries. To collate COVID-19 data, a website 'http://www.covid19-sdmc.org/' has been created by the SAARC Disaster Management Centre. Furthermore, India has developed an electronic platform called the 'SAARC COVID-19 Information Exchange Platform (COINEX)' accessible to all the SAARC countries.

STATISTICAL ANALYSIS

As of 6th November 2020, the SAARC member states have reported a total number of 9,417,660 positive cases, and out of that, 8,674,024 have been recovered, whereas 140,584 faced death (Source: Worldometer). The highest number of cases has been reported in India (8,411,724), followed by Pakistan (340,251), Bangladesh (213,254), Nepal (182,923), Afghanistan (41,935), the Maldives (11,893), Sri Lanka (12,970), and the lowest in Bhutan (358). Amongst the SAARC member states, India has the highest population, which can justify the maximum number of cases in the country. Fig. (2) shows the mortality rate, total tests, cases per million profiles, and recovery percentage for all the 8 SAARC countries.

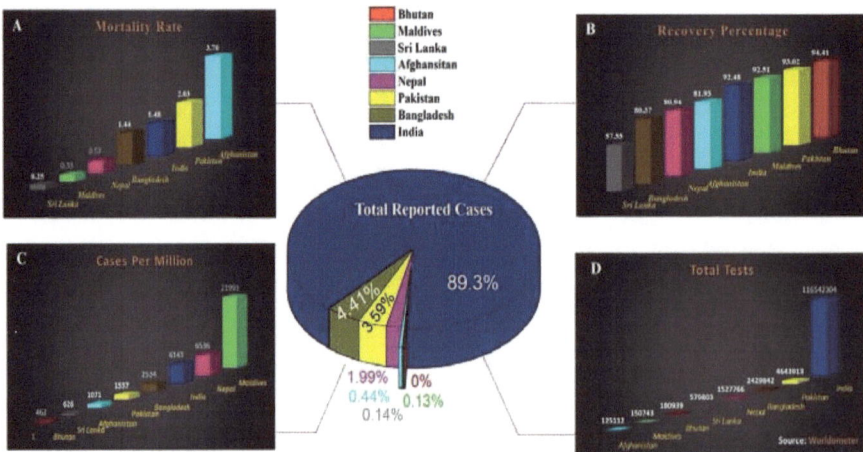

Fig. (2). Data compilation from the total reported cases- **A)** Mortality rate **B)** Total tests **C)** Cases per million profiles, and **D)** Recovery percentage (Source: Worldometer) for all the 8 SAARC countries till 6th November, 2020.

The number of deaths has been found to be continuously increasing in near geometric progression with the rise in the number of cases for each country except for Afghanistan, which showed an abrupt increase in the mortality rate. No death was recorded in Bhutan, and the first death due to COVID-19 was reported in the Maldives on 1ˢᵗ May 2020.

In India, the jump in the coronavirus cases may be linked to the public gathering in sect by Tablighi Jamaat that occurred on 13ᵗʰ March 2020, at Nizamuddin, Delhi, India. The partial lockdown in Pakistan at the initial stage of coronavirus followed by the arrival of pilgrims from Iran are the prime factors that cultivated and propagated COVID-19 disease in the country. The lowest recovery rate in Bangladesh can be reasoned based on its low testing rate and the non-availability of the appropriate treatment in most of the designed hospitals of the country. According to the Dhaka Tribune report, a limited scale of diagnosis and inadequate kits made the government find only critical cases at an early stage of COVID-19.

SAARC RESPONSE AGAINST COVID-19

To fight against COVID-19, SAARC nations are continuously making efforts to prevent the spread of the pandemic. The major initiatives by the SAARC countries have been elaborated as:

Bhutan Government has designed an intelligent integrated system (based on the latest technology) to monitor the real-time situation in the country.

In *India*, the "Aarogya Setu" App has been launched by the Central Government in 11 languages to disseminate awareness among citizens of the country about Covid-19."Lifeline Udan" flights are also operating in India to transport essential medical shipments of around 790 tonnes to the remote parts of the country during the lockdown period. India has launched "COVID KATHA", a multimedia guide on COVID 19 for mass awareness (Source:pib.gov.in). The Indian Government has announced a stimulus plan of $22.6 billion, direct cash transfer to poor women and senior citizens, free food grain, and cooking gas during the lockdown period (Source: Economic Times). The Defence Institute of Advanced Technology aided by DRDO has developed a microwave sterilizer called "ATULYA" to disintegrate the virus by differential heating in the range of 560 to 600 °C temperatures (Source: pib.gov.in). Under the Vande Bharat Mission, the repatriation of Indians has started from different countries like Bhutan, UAE, Singapore, Bangladesh, UK, USA, Canada, *etc.* and presently, it has entered into the fifth phase of the mission. Over 20 lakh of Indian citizens have returned since 7ᵗʰ May 2020.

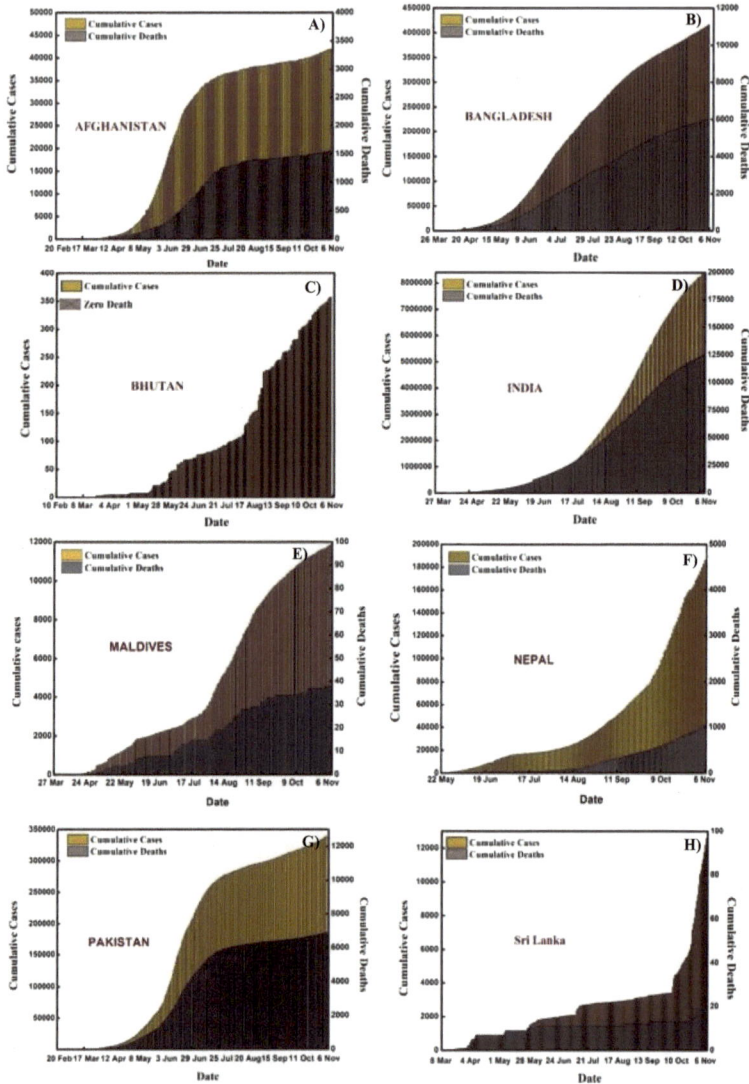

Fig. (3). shows the rise in the number of cumulative cases and deaths with each passing day starting from the onset till 6th November 2020 for all the 8 SAARC countries. A rapid increase in the number of COVID-19 cases has been found in the SAARC nations. However, the earlier imposition of lockdown in SAARC nations where the movement of people was strictly restricted happened as soon as the positive cases started to increase. The pandemic is in the community transmission stage. In contrast to the current situation, the total number of cases cannot be predicted accurately from the data given by countries to various sources (like World Bank, ECDC) because of a lower number of testing in SAARC countries. The Maldives, Bhutan, and India have tested only 29.21%, 24%, and 8.61% of their population, respectively, while other SAARC countries have tested less than 3%. Even though the number of tests is highest in India, *i.e.*, 116.54 million, still the number is very less if we compare it to the total population of the country. Limited developed hospitals, lower testing rates, lack of awareness among citizens, medical equipment are other causes associated with the spreading of coronavirus in SAARC Nations.

In *Afghanistan*, the Government has allocated about USD 25 million to deal with COVID-19. Several efforts like awareness campaigns, creation of emergency, and sectorial committees, the establishment of specific areas for the quarantines in Kabul, and screening at the airports have been made by the Ministry of Public Health in Afghanistan. Ministry of Health and Education of Afghanistan has suspended all schooling as well as restricted "Persian New Year" celebrations to fight against the Coronavirus [2].

To fight the pandemic, *Pakistan* is also under self-quarantine and the Pakistan Government has announced a relief package of $40 per month for around 7 million daily wage workers [3].

A project named "*Maldives* COVID-19 Emergency Response and Health Systems Preparedness" worth $7.3 million has been approved by the World Bank's Board of Executive Directors to help the country to prevent and detect the COVID-19 pandemic (Source: World Bank).

In *Nepal*, limited coordination among health care management stakeholders, shortage of medical supplies, testing kits, and poor reporting are the major challenges to be tackled in this pandemic [4]. India has gifted 23 tons of essential medicines to Nepal in COVID -19 crisis. There is a need for proper training through multifaceted strategies, reporting, regular monitoring, feedbacks, staffing, and beds to fight COVID-19 in Nepal.

Sri Lanka has set up a "National Operation Centre for the prevention of COVID-19 Outbreak" led by Army wing against COVID-19 battle and assisting in contact tracing to running quarantine centers. High-risk areas of Sri Lanka have been identified and brought under lockdown. Stimulus packages have been announced by the Government to prevent the financial crisis. Sri Lanka will be entering into a Bilateral Currency Swap Agreement worth $400 million with Reserve Bank of India to ensure financial stability amid COVID-19 pandemic (Source: The Hindu).

To fight the COVID-19 escalation in Bangladesh, Prime Minister Sheikh Hasina has announced a massive stimulus package of 727 billion Takas to counter adverse effects of COVID-19 pandemic.

Together, to combat the COVID-19 crisis, SAARC nations have jointly contributed to the COVID-19 emergency fund (except the announcements of the strict lockdown, stimulus economic packages, *etc.*) as shown below in Table **1**.

Table 1. COVID-19 emergency fund by SAARC Nations (Source:http://www.covid19-sdmc.org/).

Country	Contribution in COVID- 19 Emergency Fund (USD)
Afghanistan	1,000,000
Bangladesh	1,500,000
Bhutan	100,000
India	10,000,000
Maldives	200,000
Nepal	831,393.45
Pakistan	3,000,000 (proposal made from SAARC Secretariat)
Sri Lanka	5,000,000

MEDICATIONS AND VACCINES DEVELOPMENT

Recently numerous drugs have been utilized in the treatment for COVID-19, mainly including antiviral drugs like Remdesivir, Lopinavir, *etc.* (as tabulated in Table **2**).

Table 2. Recent drugs under testing for efficacy against COVID-19.

Drug	Type	Structure	Virus	Phase	Ref.
Niclosamide	Antiviral		SARS-CoV-1, MERS-CoV	Proven efficacy against some coronaviruses	[5, 6]
Arbidol	Antiviral		SARS-CoV-1, SARS-CoV-2	Proven efficacy against coronaviruses	[7]
Ivermectin	Antiviral, Antiparasitic		HIV-1, DENV1-4, VEEV, Influenza, SARS-CoV-2	Proven efficacy	[8]

(Table 2) contd.....

Drug	Type	Structure	Virus	Phase	Ref.
Lianhuaqingwen [Emodin]	Antiviral		SARS-CoV-2, Influenza Viruses	Proven efficacy	[9]
Oleoylethanolamide	Anti-Inflamatory, Immune modulator		COVID-19	Clinical Trials	[10]
Mutian®X	Antiviral	Combination of 5 or 6 drugs	Feline coronavirus (FCoV),	Clinical Trials	[11]
Remdesivir [GS-5734) and GS-441524	Antiviral		SARSCoV, MERS-CoV, filoviruses, paramyxoviruses	Proven efficacy against Coronaviruses	[12, 13]
Lopinavir, Emetine, and Homoharringtonine	Antiviral		SARS-CoV-1, MERS CoV, filoviruses, paramyxoviruses	Proven efficacy, Clinical trials for COVID-19	[14]
Ritonavir	Antiviral		SARS-CoV-2	Proven efficacy against Coronaviruses	[15]
Vitamin C	Anticancer, anti-viral properties		Immunity Booster	Proven anticancer and antiviral properties	[16]

(Table 2) contd.....

Drug	Type	Structure	Virus	Phase	Ref.
Ibuprofen	Antipyretic, Pain killer			Harmful effect while treating COVID-19	[17]
Favipiravir	Antiviral		COVID-19, Mammalian, avian boronaviruses	Clinical Trials	[18, 19]
Convalescent Plasma	Antiviral		SARS-CoV-2	Proven efficacy.	[20]
Molnupiravir (EIDD-2801)	Antiviral		SARS-CoV-2	Proven efficacy.	[21]

Across the world, all the health researchers and scientists are working hard to develop an effective vaccine against the SARS-CoV-2 virus. Currently, there are more than 150 vaccines in the clinical phase trials. For instance, the Oxford-AstraZeneca vaccine has shown positive results as a suitable vaccine to combat the COVID-19 pandemic. The vaccine was able to generate a strong immune response by producing antibodies and T-cells [22]. Oxford's vaccine is already in phase III clinical trials. Moreover, the Serum Institute of India has got the approval to start phase II/III trials of Oxford's vaccine (marketed as Covishield) in India on a large scale. Serum Institute of India has already proposed to deliver 300 million doses of Covishield by end of this year at a very low price. Apart from this, Moderna, US is developing an mRNA-based vaccine named mRNA-1273 which is in its third phase of clinical trials. Also, Novavax (USA) has entered into the third phase of clinical trials with a nanoparticle-based vaccine NVX-CoV2373.

Russia has approved two coronavirus vaccines namely: Sputnik V and EpiVacCorona without even phase 3 clinical trials. Moreover, China has also developed a recombinant vaccine Ad5-nCoV which is in the final phase of clinical trials. Sinovac Research and Development, Bejing, China has developed a vaccine candidate CoronaVac which is already in its final phase of clinical trials.

NVX-CoV2373, another promising vaccine candidate, is in clinical phase I trial. It has been developed by Novavax (America) and has shown a positive immune response. The vaccine is reportedly generating antibodies and neutralizing the SARS-CoV-2 virus in 100% of volunteers [23]. Novavax has licensed Serum

Institute of India to produce 1 billion doses of the vaccine for India and lower-middle-income countries.

Bharat Biotech India is developing India's first indigenous COVID-19 vaccine in collaboration with ICMR-NIV. The vaccine is still in phase III clinical trials.

Among the SAARC Nations, India has emerged as a leading runner for testing and trials of drugs and vaccines against coronavirus. Scientists of the Indian Institute of Technology, Jodhpur have explored the neuro invasive nature of the SARS CoV 2 virus and highlighted that loss of taste and smell of infected patients makes their central nervous system and the underlying structures in the brain more susceptible to viral infections with distressing effects (Source: pib.gov.in). Few exemplary medications under trial are discussed below:

Sepsivac

Sepsivac Immunotherapy Treatment, which is used for the management of sepsis and liver cirrhosis, is going to be tested for critically ill COVID-19 patients by the Council of Scientific and Industrial Research (CSIR). This drug is being produced with the help of Cadila Pharmaceuticals. Sepsivac drug is an immunomodulator that modulates the immune system in order to prevent it from cytokine storm and cytokine storm has been reported as one of the major factors responsible for the killing of COVID-19 patients [24] (Source: The Hindu).

AYUSH-64 and other Ayurveda Medicines

In India, the Ministry of AYUSH, ICMR, and CSIR will conduct trials on anti-malaria medicine AYUSH-64 as a potential candidate against COVID-19. Along with AYUSH-64, the trials will be conducted by employing other Ayurvedic herbs such as Ashwagandha, Guduchi, and Mulethi (Source: The Print). Use of Chawayanprash, Ashwagandha, Guduchi Ghana vati has been recommended for high-risk individuals under the Indian National Clinical Management Protocol. This protocol is based on Ayurveda and Yoga for the management of COVID-19. An ayurvedic neutraceutical Reginmune has also shown effective results for the treatment of COVID-19. Dalmia healthcare has started clinical trials of a polyherbal medicine, Astha-15 due to its efficacy and effectiveness against COVID-19. In a recent case study on herbo-mineral drugs (Siddha medicine) has shown a successful reduction in COVID-19 progression within 10 days of infection.

Mycobacterium w (MW) Vaccine

MW vaccine is an anti-leprosy vaccine that was recently tested by PGIMER, Chandigarh, India against six COVID-19 patients. A dose of 0.3 mL has shown promising results against COVID-19. Since the sample size was small (only 6 patients) CSIR will conduct a trial on a large scale for further study (Source: India Today).

Convalescent Plasma Therapy

It is a very old traditional therapy that was used to treat flu when there were no vaccines. Phase 1 studies on COVID-19 have shown that this therapy may turn effective in the treatment of Coronavirus. After being successfully used in Delhi for curing one patient, Bengaluru and Karnataka are ready to test the therapy on a large scale (Source: Indo-Asian News Service).

COVID-19: EFFECT ON SAARC ECONOMY

Apart from the irrevocable loss to society, the global economy has been demobilized by COVID-19. In order to combat the spread of this pandemic to a massive scale, all member countries of SAARC were in complete lockdown. All sectors such as the education system, aviation, hotels, all types of retail trade, tourism, *etc.* were suspended with special exemption given to sectors serving mankind. But the costs of lockdowns have already been huge and will further deepen if they result in inescapable health treatments, dropouts from school, and permanent closure of businesses. With the complete lockdown of countries, the GDP of each country (per month) has already incurred a loss of ~2% points in the annual GDP growth [25].

According to World Trade Organization (WTO) and Organization for Economic Cooperation and Development (OECD) reports, the economic shock of COVID - 19 is going to be fatal for the global economy, similar to the conditions which prevailed in the year 2008-2009 during the global financial emergency. As per UN DESA's World Economic Forecasting Model, in the worst scenario, the world economy can contract by 0.9% in 2020.

Hence, the World Bank Group is quickly taking an action to help the countries to strengthen their pandemic response, better public health interventions, and helping the private sectors by deploying up to $ 160 billion financial support over the next 15 months. However, different reports have come forth in which the effect of COVID-19 has been reflected on the GDP of all countries,

• The Indian Government estimation indicates that the real estate, professional, and financial services are going to largely hit during the lockdown period.

• The World Bank report indicated that Maldivian's economy will take the greatest hit among SAARC nations, contracting between -13 to -8.5%.

• Pakistan may fall into recession by the impact of COVID-19 and GDP might shrink in between the range of -2.2 to -1.3% (first time in the past 68 years) (Source: World Bank).

• According to the Asian Development Outlook (ADO) reports, Pakistan will "struggle this year with *double-digit inflation*". Pakistan is among countries like the Maldives, Sri Lanka, and Afghanistan, where GDP for the 2020 year is in negative territory (Source: Council of Foreign Relations).

• Afghanistan's economic growth was 2.9% in 2019, but in 2020, it is estimated to be contracted in the range of -5.9 to -3.8%.

• Bhutan's economy GDP growth projected to be declining in the range of 2.2 to 2.9%.

Table **3** shows the falls in GDP of SAARC countries estimated by the World Bank.

Table 3. Real GDP in market price given by the World Bank (Source: World Bank).

Period	Country	2019 (Estimated in %)	2020 (Forecast in %)
December - December	Afghanistan	2.9	-5.9 to -3.8
July-June	Bangladesh	8.2	2.0 to 3.0
July-June	Bhutan	3.9	2.2 to 2.9
April-March	India	6.1	4.8 to 5.0
January-December	Maldives	5.2	-13.0 to -8.5
mid July-mid July	Nepal	7.1	1.5 to 2.8
July-June	Pakistan	3.3	-2.2 to -1.3
January-December	Sri Lanka	2.6	-3.0 to -0.5

COVID-19: IMPACT ON SAARC ENVIRONMENT

While an unusual outburst of lethal COVID-19 has proved catastrophic to the world by dwindling countries' economies due to the lockdown imposed on global production, consumption, and employment. A rapid decrease in the pollution level *i.e.*, NO_2 and CO_2 emissions seem to be another positive half of the pandemic.

Climate experts using the **Global Carbon Project, 2020** predicted that greenhouse gases may drop to unexpected proportions in the coming years [26]. However, this effect is limited only for a short period, as soon as the pandemic will end or lockdown will be lifted, a sudden surge in economic activities will again leave the world in a vast sea of pollution.

We have forgotten the amount of waste which has been generated due to this pandemic. Due to the quarantine policies, the production of organic waste (generated by households daily) and inorganic waste (online food packing based waste) has massively increased around the world. The amount of biomedical waste (contaminated masks, gloves, used syringes, and medications) has risen substantially to another level. Hand sanitizer's empty bottles along with solid tissue papers are ending up into gigantic medical waste in the environment [27]. The face masks are made up of liquid-resistant plastic-based materials that are long-lasting which are later resulting in a landfill. To combat the COVID-19, the general public has started wearing surgical masks as a preventive measure. When such a large number of people start wearing the mask, one pair of gloves, and use hand sanitizer, the amount of created garbage is going to be significant.

Among SAARC nations, India generated nearly 559 tonnes per day of biomedical waste in 2017 which is expected to increase substantially during this pandemic.

Pakistan's hospitals have generated almost 240 metric tons of medical waste on a per-day basis and it is gigantic (almost 6 times as were before) in this crisis without proper management to dump the harmful trashes.

In Afghanistan, Kabul Municipality, the only government agency to deal with municipal waste does not have a proper waste management system.

In Sri Lanka, the raw sewage is directly discharged into rivers by the factories (Source: Monogabay News & Inspiration from Nature's Frontline).

Overall, In SAARC nations, medical waste has been increasing due to the COVID -19 outbreak which can also act as a carrier for the pandemic in the future. Therefore, the Governments have chalk down strategies like the Indian Government's Central Pollution Control Board (CPCB) has issued guidelines including the usage of double-layered bags and color-coded bins for the management of waste generated during the diagnostics and treatment of COVID-19 patients (Source: Economic Times). Also, responsibility is given to a person (operating in sewage treatment) to clarify the general waste from the quarantine homes, masks, gloves, and other medical waste. Fig. (**4**) shows the positive and negative impact of COVID-19 on the environment.

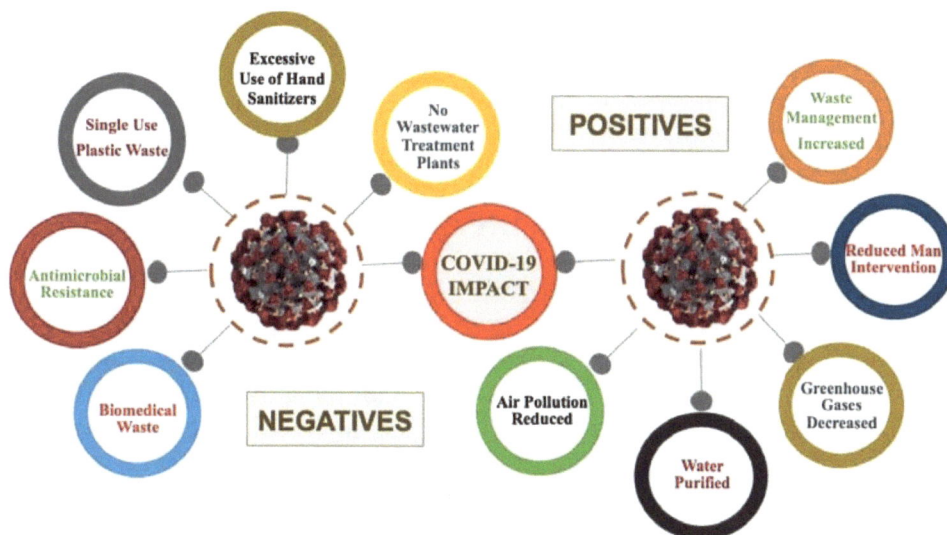

Fig. (4). COVID-19 Impact on Environment .

Due to the pandemic spread, many countries have stopped the waste recycling process that has created a hazardous effect on the environment (as recycling is an effective way to prevent pollution and conserve natural resources). Especially the countries of SAARC nations that include developing nations with minimal medical facility and biomedical waste handling practices. The lack of wastewater treatment plants in SAARC countries leads to the release of all these harmful wastes into the environment.

Apart from the biomedical waste, the use of single-use plastic during the COVID-19 pandemic has increased suddenly. While most countries were imposing a ban on single-use plastic before COVID-19, now the usage has increased tremendously. People find a single-use plastic to be an easier and safer alternative in this crisis time. SAARC countries are ranked 3rd in the world for generating a staggering amount of 334 million metric tonnes of solid waste every year.

Moreover, to battle the COVID-19, several antiviral drugs have been tested and recommended for use without a prior detailed study on their fate in the environment. As most of these drugs are not fully metabolized by the human body, they make their way finally into the water or soil [28]. This has eventually increased the amount of organic pharmaceutical waste in the environment. A majority of pharmaceutical drugs are lipophilic and they remain as such in water for a long period. This could lead to an increase in antimicrobial resistance of drugs, which already is a serious problem in today's world. A large number of coronaviruses are present in birds which have not been fatal for humans yet [29]. But if birds or animals will be exposed to these pharmaceutical antimicrobials, they may develop antimicrobial resistance and if such a virus makes a future jump to humans, the results could be devastating.

COVID-19: EFFECT ON EDUCATION SECTOR

The widespread COVID-19 has led to the closure of Educational Institutions almost everywhere in the World but the education sector has got severely affected in SAARC. Most of the education in the SAARC nations is given through an offline classroom system. To combat the situation all the Governments of SAARC nations have recently taken a major shift from a Classical offline mode of education to Online learning programs by undergoing digitization of all the resources. However, it requires plenty of time to transform the classical offline classroom into an e-learning based education system even in the Post COVID-19 period. Apart from ensuring the safety of students by complete closure and suspension of classes, the Government has been continuously issuing guidelines and notifications to the educational institutions to deliver effective education to students for capacity building of young minds. By engaging in innovative teaching approaches, the educational institutions have been taking care of the students who are affected by disease-associated fear and pressure by providing professional psychological services to them.

FUTURE COURSE OF ACTION

The rampant spread of COVID-19 has led to a failure of the contemporary world order. It will be better if we examine the coronavirus battle strategies of different countries like South Korea, Japan, Singapore, *etc.* in order to contain the virus successfully. With the collaboration of the scientific research community, the knowledge gained from the spread of disease in other countries can be shared and a successful strategy can be formulated to battle against the virus by SAARC nations.

The best way to mitigate this biological threat is that everyone makes collective efforts and maintain proper social distancing and proper coordination with the Government. From time to time guidelines issued by the respective Governments should be strictly followed. Fig. (**5**) shows the method to mitigate COVID-19 pandemic. Flattening of the peak can be achieved by the following steps: Social distancing, use of masks, isolation, and quarantine, and most importantly, increasing the testing rate. To restore the economic and social life, there is a prerequisite need for smart designing of policies, targeting the lower-risk segments of the population to return in the daily activities while protecting the higher-risk ones. WHO, World Bank, IMF are providing financial help to poor and developing nations to fight against the pandemic. Government and National banks of respective countries have taken steps to infuse money in the global market to mitigate economic distress. Building healthcare system capacity and following WHO guidelines strictly will surely decrease the impact of the virus on SAARC Nations.

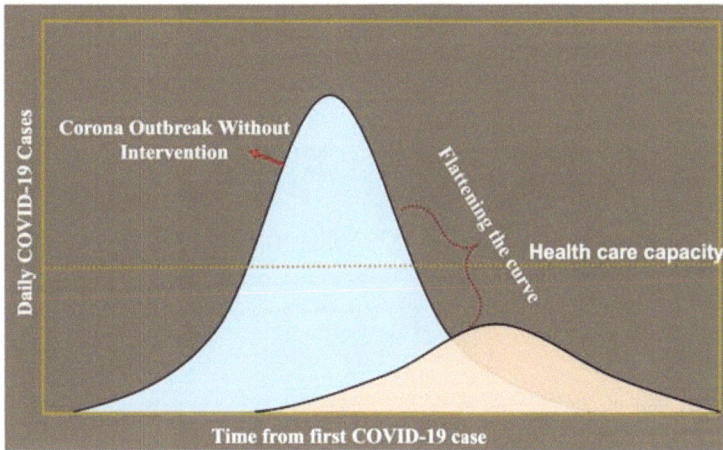

Fig. (5).   Goals of community mitigation can be achieved by delaying outbreak peak in order to decompressing the burden on hospitals/infrastructure and diminish overall cases and health impacts.

CONCLUSION

Since SAARC nations make 21% of world's population, the fate of COVID-19 in these nations has a huge impact at global level. To fight against COVID-19, SAARC nations are continuously making efforts to prevent the spread of this pandemic. However, despite the implementations like lockdowns, closure of governmental and non-governmental organisations, social-distancing, *etc.* the number of COVID-19 cases and deaths has increased tremendously in SAARC countries. Apart from the irrevocable loss to the society, the global economy, environment and educational sector have been drastically affected by COVID-19. Although numerous drugs have been utilized in the treatment for COVID-19 and >150 vaccines are under clinical phase trials but the virus is still haunting the society.

CONSENT FOR PUBLICATION

Not applicable.

CONFLICT OF INTEREST

Declared none.

ACKNOWLEDGEMENTS

Surinder Kumar Mehta is grateful to the CSIR project grant (Sanction No. 01(2951)/18/EMR-II). Jyoti Rathee is thankful to UGC (No. F.16-6(DEC.2016)/2017 NET) for the stipend. Amit Kumar acknowledges DST-INSPIRE (DST/INSPIRE Fellowship/2018/IF180772) for fellowship.

REFERENCES

[1]   Du L, He Y, Zhou Y, Liu S, Zheng BJ, Jiang S. The spike protein of SARS-CoV--a target for vaccine and therapeutic development. Nat Rev Microbiol 2009; 7(3): 226-36.
[http://dx.doi.org/10.1038/nrmicro2090] [PMID: 19198616]

[2]   Shah J, Karimzadeh S, Al-ahdal TMA, Mousavi SH, Zahid SU, Huy NT. Correspondence COVID-19 : the current situation in Afghanistan. Lancet Glob Heal 2020; (20): 19-20.

[3]   Nafees M, Khan F. Pakistan's Response to COVID-19 Pandemic and Efficacy of Quarantine and Partial Lockdown : A Review. Electron J Gen Med 2020; 17(2): 17-20.

[4]   Asim M, Sathian B, van Teijlingen E, Mekkodathil A, Subramanya SH, Simkhada P. COVID-19 pandemic: Public health implications in Nepal. Nepal J Epidemiol 2020; 10(1): 817-20.
[http://dx.doi.org/10.3126/nje.v10i1.28269] [PMID: 32257511]

[5]   Wen CC, Kuo YH, Jan JT, et al. Specific plant terpenoids and lignoids possess potent antiviral activities against severe acute respiratory syndrome coronavirus. J Med Chem 2007; 50(17): 4087-95.
[http://dx.doi.org/10.1021/jm070295s] [PMID: 17663539]

[6]   Xu J, Shi PY, Li H, Zhou J. Broad Spectrum Antiviral Agent Niclosamide and Its Therapeutic Potential. ACS Infect Dis 2020; 6(5): 909-15.
[http://dx.doi.org/10.1021/acsinfecdis.0c00052] [PMID: 32125140]

[7]   Zhu Z, Lu Z, Xu T, et al. Arbidol monotherapy is superior to lopinavir/ritonavir in treating COVID-19. J Infect 2020; 81(1): e21-3.
[http://dx.doi.org/10.1016/j.jinf.2020.03.060] [PMID: 32283143]

[8]   Caly L, Druce JD, Catton MG, Jans DA, Wagstaff KM. The FDA-approved drug ivermectin inhibits the replication of SARS-CoV-2 in vitro. Antiviral Res 2020; 178104787
[http://dx.doi.org/10.1016/j.antiviral.2020.104787] [PMID: 32251768]

[9]   Runfeng L, Yunlong H, Jicheng H, et al. Lianhuaqingwen exerts anti-viral and anti-inflammatory activity against novel coronavirus (SARS-CoV-2). Pharmacol Res 2020; 156104761
[http://dx.doi.org/10.1016/j.phrs.2020.104761] [PMID: 32205232]

[10]   Ghaffari S, Roshanravan N, Tutunchi H, Ostadrahimi A, Pouraghaei M, Kafil B. Oleoylethanolamide, A Bioactive Lipid Amide, as A Promising Treatment Strategy for Coronavirus/COVID-19. Arch Med Res 2020; 51(5): 464-7.
[http://dx.doi.org/10.1016/j.arcmed.2020.04.006] [PMID: 32327293]

[11]   Addie DD, Curran S, Bellini F, et al. Oral Mutian®X stopped faecal feline coronavirus shedding by naturally infected cats. Res Vet Sci 2020; 130: 222-9.
[http://dx.doi.org/10.1016/j.rvsc.2020.02.012] [PMID: 32220667]

[12]   Amirian ES, Levy JK. Current knowledge about the antivirals remdesivir (GS-5734) and GS-441524 as therapeutic options for coronaviruses. One Health 2020; 9100128
[http://dx.doi.org/10.1016/j.onehlt.2020.100128] [PMID: 32258351]

[13]   Cao YC, Deng QX, Dai SX. Remdesivir for severe acute respiratory syndrome coronavirus 2 causing COVID-19: An evaluation of the evidence. Travel Med Infect Dis 2020; 35101647 [http://dx.doi.org/10.1016/j.tmaid.2020.101647] [PMID: 32247927]

[14]   Choy KT, Wong AYL, Kaewpreedee P, *et al.* Remdesivir, lopinavir, emetine, and homoharringtonine inhibit SARS-CoV-2 replication *in vitro* . Antiviral Res 2020; 178104786 [http://dx.doi.org/10.1016/j.antiviral.2020.104786] [PMID: 32251767]

[15]   Bhatnagar T, Murhekar MV, Soneja M, *et al.* Lopinavir/ritonavir combination therapy amongst symptomatic coronavirus disease 2019 patients in India: Protocol for restricted public health emergency use. Indian J Med Res 2020; 151(2 & 3): 184-9. [PMID: 32362644]

[16]   Boretti A, Banik BK. Intravenous vitamin C for reduction of cytokines storm in acute respiratory distress syndrome. PharmaNutrition 2020; 12100190 [http://dx.doi.org/10.1016/j.phanu.2020.100190] [PMID: 32322486]

[17]   Day M. Covid-19: ibuprofen should not be used for managing symptoms, say doctors and scientists. BMJ 2020; 368: m1086. [http://dx.doi.org/10.1136/bmj.m1086] [PMID: 32184201]

[18]   Harismah K, Mirzaei M. Favipiravir: Structural Analysis and Activity against COVID-19. Adv J Chem Sec B: Na Pro Med Chem 2020; 2(2): 55-60.

[19]   Tokunaga T, Yamamoto Y, Sakai M, Tomonaga K, Honda T. Antiviral activity of favipiravir (T-705) against mammalian and avian bornaviruses. Antiviral Res 2017; 143: 237-45. [http://dx.doi.org/10.1016/j.antiviral.2017.04.018] [PMID: 28465146]

[20]   Shen C, Wang Z, Zhao F, *et al.* Treatment of 5 critically ill patients with COVID-19 with convalescent plasma. JAMA 2020; 323(16): 1582-9. [http://dx.doi.org/10.1001/jama.2020.4783] [PMID: 32219428]

[21]   Wahl A, Gralinski L, Johnson C, *et al.* Acute SARS-CoV-2 Infection is Highly Cytopathic, Elicits a Robust Innate Immune Response and is Efficiently Prevented by EIDD-2801. Research Square 2020.

[22]   Folegatti PM, Ewer KJ, Aley PK, *et al.* Safety and immunogenicity of the ChAdOx1 nCoV-19 vaccine against SARS-CoV-2: a preliminary report of a phase 1/2, single-blind, randomised controlled trial. Lancet 2020; 396(10249): 467-78. [http://dx.doi.org/10.1016/S0140-6736(20)31604-4] [PMID: 32702298]

[23]   Keech C, Albert G, Reed O, Neal S, Plested JS, Zhu M, *et al.* First-in-Human Trial of a SARS CoV 2 Recombinant Spike Protein Nanoparticle Vaccine. bioxRxiv [http://dx.doi.org/10.1101/2020.08.05.20168435]

[24]   Mehta P, McAuley DF, Brown M, Sanchez E, Tattersall RS, Manson JJ. COVID-19: consider cytokine storm syndromes and immunosuppression. Lancet 2020; 395(10229): 1033-4. [http://dx.doi.org/10.1016/S0140-6736(20)30628-0] [PMID: 32192578]

[25]   Chakraborty I, Maity P. COVID-19 outbreak: Migration, effects on society, global environment and prevention. Sci Total Environ 2020; 728138882 [http://dx.doi.org/10.1016/j.scitotenv.2020.138882] [PMID: 32335410]

[26]   Zambrano-Monserrate MA, Ruano MA, Sanchez-Alcalde L. Indirect effects of COVID-19 on the environment. Sci Total Environ 2020; 728138813 [http://dx.doi.org/10.1016/j.scitotenv.2020.138813] [PMID: 32334159]

[27]   Saadat S, Rawtani D, Hussain CM. Environmental perspective of COVID-19. Sci Total Environ 2020; 728138870 [http://dx.doi.org/10.1016/j.scitotenv.2020.138870] [PMID: 32335408]

[28]   Nannou C, Ofrydopoulou A, Evgenidou E, Heath D, Heath E, Lambropoulou D. Antiviral drugs in aquatic environment and wastewater treatment plants: A review on occurrence, fate, removal and

ecotoxicity. Sci Total Environ 2020; 699134322
[http://dx.doi.org/10.1016/j.scitotenv.2019.134322] [PMID: 31678880]

[29] Miłek J, Blicharz-Domańska K. Coronaviruses in avian species – review with focus on epidemiology and diagnosis in wild birds. J Vet Res (Pulawy) 2018; 62(3): 249-55.
[http://dx.doi.org/10.2478/jvetres-2018-0035] [PMID: 30584600]

CHAPTER 3

Neutralizing Antibody-Based Therapies against COVID-19

Hilal Çalık[1], Rabia Yılmaz[1], Hatice Feyzan Ay[1], Betül Mutlu[1] and Rabia Çakır-Koç[1,2,*]

[1] *Yıldız Technical University, Faculty of Chemical and Metallurgical Engineering, Department of Bioengineering, Istanbul, Turkey*

[2] *Health Institutes of Turkey (TUSEB), Turkey Biotechnology Institute, Istanbul, Turkey*

Abstract: The novel coronavirus infection (COVID-19) that emerged from Wuhan, China in December 2019 caused a global health crisis. With confirmed cases worldwide exceeding 40 million and continuing to grow, many research groups have been working to develop therapeutics and vaccines against COVID-19. In fact, some vaccine candidates are currently being tested in the clinical phase. The primary target of most of the studies is the spike glycoprotein of the SARS-CoV-2 virus, which binds to ACE2 receptors and allowing the virus entry to the host cells for the initiation of infection. Drugs such as Hydroxychloroquine and Favipiravir only aim to minimize symptoms but cause severe side effects in patients. On the other hand, neutralizing antibodies represents an important strategy for the treatment of COVID-19. Therapeutic neutralizing antibodies against SARS-CoV-2 spike protein can induce antibodies to block virus binding and fusion, thus inhibiting viral infection. Clinical studies show that antibodies obtained from plasma of recovered patients can improve prognosis and increase the survival rate. However, obtaining a high amount of plasma-based antibodies is a major problem in practice, therefore there is an urgent need to develop and produce reliable, high-yield, and specific antibodies against COVID-19. Instead of convalescent plasma therapy, monoclonal antibodies, and other antibody-based therapies such as IgY antibodies, camelid antibodies/nanobodies offer a promising alternative. In this chapter, a perspective on antibody-based approaches currently developed against SARS-CoV-2 by given some fundamental knowledge about these neutralizing antibodies and their potential for the treatment of COVID-19 is presented.

Keywords: Camelid antibodies, Convalescent plasma therapy, IgY antibodies, Monoclonal antibody, Neutralizing antibodies, SARS-CoV-2.

* **Corresponding Author Rabia Çakır-Koç:** Yıldız Technical University, Faculty of Chemical and Metallurgical Engineering, Department of Bioengineering, Istanbul, Turkey and Health Institutes of Turkey (TUSEB), Turkey Biotechnology Institute, Istanbul, Turkey; Tel: +90 212 383 4626; Fax: +90 212 383 4625; E-mail: rabiacakir@gmail.com

Jean-Marc Sabatier (Ed.)
All rights reserved-© 2021 Bentham Science Publishers

INTRODUCTION

The new coronavirus, SARS-CoV-2, which emerged in Wuhan, China's Hubei province, in late December 2019, spread to many countries in a short time and became an international pandemic affecting the whole world. According to the World Health Organization, the pandemic affected over 40 million people in the world and caused the death of more than 1 million people.

COVID-19 can cause different clinical manifestations ranging from asymptomatic disease to fatal disease [1]. The disease may initially show little or no symptoms. Typical symptoms of COVID-19 are fever, sore throat, cough, fatigue, shortness of breath, weakness, and muscular pain, however, new symptoms are reported every day such as loss of the sense of smell because the clinical outcomes of the disease have been clarified yet [2]. The disease is usually transmitted through respiratory droplets, hands, or surfaces contaminated by the virus and the incubation period of the disease is generally between 3-14 days [3].

Experimental and clinical studies of antiviral drugs (such as remdesivir, chloroquine, hydroxychloroquine, ritonavir), convalescent plasma transfusion, and vaccine formulations against COVID-19 disease have been ongoing. The safety of some antiviral drugs such as favipiravir and remdesivir used in the treatment of the disease is not certain and clinical studies are still ongoing [4]. Another treatment option is plasma transfusion from the recovered patient, but the difficulty in obtaining plasma during recovery and limited resources (donor) make clinical application difficult [5]. Drug and vaccine studies against COVID-19 disease are a key strategy both to prevent widespread viral infection and to reduce morbidity and mortality [2].

Currently, more than 230 vaccine candidates are in pre-clinical and clinical development to prevent SARS-CoV-2 infection [6]. On December 11, 2020, the first vaccine for Covid19 disease, the Pfizer-BioNTech COVID-19 (BNT162b2) mRNA vaccine (Pfizer, Inc; Philadelphia, Pennsylvania) had been approved by the Food and Drug Administration (FDA) with Emergency Use Authorization (EUA) [7]. Moderna COVID-19 (mRNA-1273) vaccine (ModernaTX, Inc; Cambridge, Massachusetts) is the second mRNA vaccine approved by the Food and Drug Administration (FDA) with Emergency Use Authorization (EUA) on December 18, 2020 [8]. Also, an adenoviral vector vaccine, ChAdOx1 nCoV-19 (AZD1222), developed by a group from the University of Oxford is currently being evaluated in phase II/III efficacy trials [9]. In today's drug and vaccine studies, new molecular biotechnological methods are more preferred in order to obtain products that are therapeutically more effective with fewer side effects [10]. Since the '90s, with the development of recombinant gene technology and molecular immunology, antibodies created against various diseases *in vitro* or *in vivo* have been humanized by gene engineering. The binding kinetics of antibodies have been increased and the ability to work in coordination with the immune system in a physiological environment has been gained. Because of these developments, antibody-based therapeutic applications gain important potential in clinic studies [11]. Antibody therapy, one of the fast and effective treatment in contrast to the traditional vaccine approaches, against SARS-CoV-2 offers a promising strategy in the control of the pandemic in terms of prophylactic and therapeutic purposes.

Coronaviruses consist of 4 main protein domains structurally; the surface spike (S) glycoprotein, the membrane (M) protein, the small envelope (E) glycoprotein, and the nucleocapsid (N) protein [12]. The spike (S) glycoprotein on the surface of the SARS-CoV-2 has an important role in the viral entrance [13]. In recent studies, it has been proven that the S protein of the SARS-CoV-2 virus is more likely to bind to the ACE2 receptor than other coronavirus types which cause the new coronavirus to spread faster among humans [14]. The S1 subunit of the S protein binds to angiotensin-converting enzyme 2 (ACE2) receptors, which are commonly found in respiratory system cells. The S2 subunit of the S protein mediates the fusion of the viral membrane to the host cell membrane [1]. Thus, blocking the S protein, which has an important role in the entry of the virus into the cell, with neutralizing antibodies is one of the main strategies of antibody therapies [15]. S1 subunit, particularly the S1-RBD, S1-N-terminal domain (NTD), and S2 domain has been the main target of neutralizing antibodies due to their high functionality in infection of the virus [16].

In this chapter, a perspective on neutralizing antibody approaches based on monoclonal antibodies, convalescent plasma antibodies, IgY antibodies, and camelid antibodies and their potential for the treatment of COVID-19 are presented.

Convalescent Plasma Therapy

Immune or convalescent plasma means plasma collected from recovered individuals with high titers antibodies. Convalescent plasma contains antibodies and proteins against the pathogen. Convalescent plasma therapy (CPT) is the administration of blood plasma taken from people recovered to individuals suffering from the same disease [17, 18]. The concept of CPT was created in the 1880s against diphtheria and tetanus toxins by using antibodies obtained in the blood of actively infected animals [19, 20]. After that CPT has been used for over a century. In the early 1900s, the use of CPT for infectious diseases such as poliomyelitis, small measles, and mumps was studied [21 - 23].

In the mid-1900s, a high concentration of immunoglobulins purified from recovered human donors has provided the option of treating serious infectious diseases [24, 25]. In the following years, the development of various passive antibody therapies has allowed its use for the treatment of primary immunodeficiencies, autoimmune, and cancer diseases as well as infective diseases [26]. However, the lack of time and resources for the production of these passive antibody therapy products in emergencies such as epidemics has brought convalescent plasma therapy back to the agenda as an experimental therapeutic treatment as far as the development of effective drugs or vaccines [18].

It is thought that immune plasma/convalescent plasma therapy produces therapeutic effects in patients through various mechanisms. The most accepted mechanism is the neutralization of the pathogen with antibodies [27]. Antibodies in the plasma can bind to specific regions of the pathogen and blocking their cell entrance. In addition, other mechanisms such as stimulation of complement activation, antibody-dependent cellular cytotoxicity and/or phagocytosis might promote the therapeutic effect. Non-neutralizing antibodies in the plasma that can bind to the pathogen are also thought to contribute to prophylaxis and/or enhancement of healing by marking the pathogen for immune cells [24].

The first data on the use of CPT against coronavirus were obtained from Severe Acute Respiratory Syndrome 1 (SARS-CoV-1) outbreaks in 2003. In a retrospective, nonrandomized study, 40 SARS patients were treated with methylprednisolone and 200-400 mL CP (n = 19) and methylprednisolone alone (n = 21). Patients treated with methylprednisolone and CPT had a higher discharge rate from the hospital up to 22 days and a lower mortality rate than patients treated with drugs alone [28]. A similar non-randomized Cohort study evaluating the effectiveness of CPT with 80 SARS patients who were non-responsive to treatment with methylprednisolone demonstrated that patients who received CP before day 14 have a higher discharge rate and lower mortality rate (12.5% *versus* 17%) than the control group [29]. A study in Taiwan was reported that three patients with SARS-CoV-1 who were refractory to steroids, antivirals, and protease inhibitors have been successfully treated with a dose of 500 mL CP [30]. Another study in South Korea reported that three Middle East Respiratory Syndrome (MERS) patients with respiratory insufficiency were infused with CP at 4 different antibody titers and a serological response was reported after CP infusion with a neutralizing activity titer of 1:80 [31]. Although these studies are generally case-series including a small number of patients and lack randomization, it has only led to ideas about the positive effect of CP therapy in the treatment of various coronavirus infections.

The recent emergence of the coronavirus (COVID-19) pandemic has raised the topic of CPT again. From the experience gained from previous SARS-CoV and MERS-CoV outbreaks, it was predicted that convalescent plasma therapy could also be a good treatment option for the SARS-CoV-2 pandemic [32]. The increasing number of patients recovering with high neutralizing antibody titer makes convalescent plasma treatment an experimental therapeutic treatment option, especially for severe COVID-19 patients [32, 33]. The first application of convalescent plasma therapy for COVID-19 was carried out in China, Shen *et al.* reported that 5 COVID-19 patients who did not respond to steroid and antiviral therapy received 400 mL of CP transfusion from 5 different donors [34]. They reported that 3 days after the transfusion, 4 of 5 patients that their body temperature returned to normal and the viral load decreased and their test became negative within 12 days. Also in China, recovery plasma therapy was applied in a pilot study of 245 COVID-19 patients, and 91 patients showed improvement in terms of clinical signs and symptoms [35].

Duan *et al.* reported the results of a pilot CPT study involving 10 patients with severe COVID-19. Patients were given plasma at a 1:640 dilution of 200 mL or higher with neutralizing antibody titers and no serious adverse effects were observed [36]. All patients experienced an improvement in symptoms of fever, cough, shortness of breath, and chest pain within 1 to 3 days after transfusion. Radiological improvements were also detected in pulmonary lesions but viral load had increased in 7 patients. In another study of 6 cases of COVID-19 pneumonia in Wuhan, it has been shown that a single 200 ml dose of CP administered at a late stage resulted in viral clearance in 2 patients and radiological improvement in 5 patients [37].

In another study, the clinical progress of 25 COVID-19 patients who were received CP transfusion has been evaluated on the basis of the World Health Organization (WHO) six-point ordinal scale and laboratory parameters. On the 14th day after transfusion, it was found that 19 patients showed at least one point improvement in clinical condition [38].

In a case series, the early clinical findings of 20 hospitalized patients treated with CP were compared with 20 matched controls and patients have shown improvements according to laboratory and respiratory parameters. Also, 7 and 14-day mortality rates in patients with CP are more favorable than controls [39].

In addition to all these studies, retrospective randomized controlled studies have also been conducted. In the USA, severely ill COVID-19 patients were transfused CP containing a SARS-CoV-2 anti-spike antibody with the titer at a 1:320, then data such as supplemental oxygen requirements and survival were compared between plasma group and controls [40]. In this study, it was found that patients with severe COVID-19 treated with CP showed a better survival rate compared to control. In another multicenter controlled clinical study conducted in Iran (IRCT20200325046860N1), 115 patients were given CP and compared with the control group (n = 74) in terms of clinical findings such as the length of hospital stay and need for intubation and mortality rates. The authors reported that a total of 98 (98.2%) patients who received CP were discharged from the hospital, which was quite high compared to the discharge rate in the control group of 56 (78.7%). While 7% of the patients who received plasma treatment intubated, while this rate was 20% in the control group [41].

In a recent study in China, the effects of adding CPT to standard therapy in severe COVID-19 patients on clinical recovery time compared to standard therapy were investigated in a randomized clinical trial involving 103 patients [42]. CPT added to standard therapy was found associated with clinical improvement in severe patients between COVID-19 patients, while no statistically significant difference was found on clinical improvement within 28 days. However, the researchers have indicated that early termination of the trial may cause insufficiency to detect a clinically significant difference too.

As of today, there are 168 clinical trials currently underway in various countries (https://www.covid-trials.org/). To date, most of the studies have provided evidence to support that CPT can be used as an effective intervention in COVID-19. However, issues such as the lack of an appropriate general guideline for treatment, concerns about side effects, and the small number of donors have caused hesitation in applying this treatment widely. The Blood Regulators Network (BRN) and the World Health Organization (WHO) have recommended the use of CP in the treatment of critical patients with COVID-19.

Patients recovering with a higher neutralizing antibody titer from COVID-19 are considered as eligible donors. Based on the currently available data, it can be said that serum IgM and IgA against SARS-CoV-2 appear 5 days after symptom onset, and IgG antibodies develop and can be detected between 6-15 days after the onset of the disease [43, 44]. It has been shown that the majority of the neutralizing antibody response is associated with the IgG1 and IgG3 subclasses [45]. The eligibility criteria for a plasma donor differ between countries. According to FDA guidelines, serums should be collected from individuals who have recovered from COVID-19 whose associated symptoms completely ceased at least 14 days before donation [46]. Plasma donors should be evaluated before donation with various screening tests as antibody detection tests, and all other for routine blood donation. ABO blood group compatibility is preferred for plasma transfusion. In addition, female donors with a pregnancy history should be investigated in terms of human leukocyte antigens (HLA) antibodies [47].

Donor's plasma that meets the criteria is collected by apheresis and stored by freezing or can be applied within 6 hours. For transfusion safety, it is recommended that CP passes through the pathogen inactivation process [48]. Although the duration time of anti-SARS-CoV-2 antibodies in plasma is currently unknown, it has been found that neutralizing antibodies specific to SARS are typically found to be 2 years [49]. It is therefore thought that a suitable donor can donate about 600 ml of plasma (equivalent to almost 3 therapeutic doses) at regular intervals for at least 6 months.

Another concern limiting the use of CP is the possible side effects of treatment. The passive application of serums in the recovery period also has some known and theoretical risks such as transfusion-transmitted infections (TTI), allergic transfusion reactions such as serum sickness, transfusion-associated hyper-circulation (TACO), transfusion-associated acute lung injury (TRALI). Another risk associated with transfusion is an antibody-induced increased infection phenomenon known as antibody-dependent enhancement (ADE). ADE refers to a process in which antibodies targeting one coronavirus serotype are exacerbated by infection and disease to another viral serotype [50]. Therefore, patients treated with convalescent plasma should be closely monitored for adverse effects, particularly for evidence of inflammatory exacerbation [51].

In a comprehensive current study, the safety of healing plasma [NCT04338360] in 5000 critical hospitalized COVID-19 patients was investigated. They have reported a mortality rate of 0.3% within the first 4 hours after transfusion, and an incidence of <1% for all serious adverse events (SAE), and a 7-day mortality rate of 14.9%. Twenty-one of 36 serious adverse events reported were caused by transfusion-associated hypercirculation (TACO; n=7), transfusion-related acute lung injury (TRALI; n=11), and severe allergic transfusion reactions (n=3) [52]. In the study, which was later updated with 20000 patients, they reported that the risk of TACO was 0.18%, and the risk of severe allergic transfusion reactions and TRALI was 0.1% [53]. These current studies have provided valid evidence that CPT is safe in hospitalized patients with severe COVID-19 [53].

In addition to all these studies, systemic reviews and meta-analyses have been conducted. Two systematic reviews and meta-analysis of the efficiency of CPT for the treatment of COVID-19 reported a significant reduction in viral loads and improvement in clinical symptoms after CP transfusion to critically ill covid-19 patients [33, 54]. In a systematic review and meta-analysis of seven studies involving 5444 patients (two randomized controlled trials and five cohort studies),

Sarkar *et al.* have concluded that the use of CPT in patients with COVID-19 reduces mortality, increases viral clearance, and provides clinical improvement. These results are also consistent with the systematic review and meta-analysis results evaluating the effectiveness of CPT for SARS [55].

Although all these encouraging scientific data show that CP therapy is clinically effective and safe in COVID-19 patients, more robust evidence is needed for the definitive effectiveness of the treatment, given the size and variability of the study groups. For this, well-designed large multicenter clinical researches are urgently needed. Although CP treatment is a fast and effective treatment method that can be applied in difficult situations, it is not a permanent solution against the disease. As the efficacy of CP is largely related to the amount of antibody titers, it cannot be a sustainable source of therapy. Therefore, specific and reliable neutralizing antibodies such as monoclonal, recombinant antibodies should be developed using reverse engineering methods from antibody products derived from CP.

Monoclonal Antibody Treatment for COVID-19

In recent years, monoclonal antibodies (mAbs) are becoming important therapeutics that use in the diagnosis and treatment of many diseases. mAbs were first produced from immortal hybridoma cells obtained by fusion of myeloma cells and B lymphocytes in 1975 by Köhler and Milstein [56, 57]. mAbs have monovalent affinity since they bind to the same epitope on the target antigen. Thus, they exhibit high specificity for a single epitope, they are less likely to cross-reactivity with other proteins and become more successful in treatments [58, 59]. Nonetheless, these antibodies have high specificity but have disadvantages such as high cost and labor requirement [60]. mAbs have been developed using many different techniques, include hybridoma technology, phage and yeast display, isolation of single B-cell, and by using transgenic mice.

Hybridoma technology is based on the fusion of immortal myeloma cells with spleen cells of immunized animals. mAbs produced by this technology have homogenous with the same specificity [61]. They have four types, including murine, chimeric, humanized, and fully human. Since murin mAbs induce a human antimouse antibody (HAMA) response in humans, chimeric and humanized mAbs were developed. However, they also caused human anti-chimeric antibody (HACA), and human anti-human antibody (HAHA) responses, respectively, due to portions of mouse origin [61, 62]. The advancement of recombinant DNA technology contributes to overcome these problems by grafting the Fc and variable regions of mouse antibodies with human counterparts [63].

One of these approaches for display antibody variable regions on the surface is the phage display technique, which contains recombinant antibodies libraries cloned into bacteriophage or yeast [64]. Smith *et al.*, developed a phage display by cloning the antigen-binding sites of Ig heavy (VH) and light (VL) genes and they were created single-chain Fv (scFv) or Fab gene repertoires. Through cloning the repertoires as fusion proteins with a bacteriophage coat protein, a phage-display antibody library was developed. The phage includes functional antibody protein and thereby, panels of antibodies with the desired specificity can be selected [65, 66]. The use of transgenic animals is another alternative approach to the development of human mAbs. The mouse antibody gene is replaced by human immunoglobulin loci in these mice. Afterward, transgenic mice have immunized with the target antigen, in order to provide the specific human antibodies expression [67, 68]. The basic advantage of monoclonal antibodies obtained from transgenic mice is their high affinity [69].

Moreover, the humanization of mAbs offered a reduction in the potential of immunological response, and thus mAbs became a better and safe opportunity. In particular, the target selectivity of mAbs prevents unnecessary exposure of drugs in non-target organs [70]. mAbs are used to treat most diseases, especially cancer and immune disorders [71].

Viral infections can be prevented by targeting their viral entry into host cells by antibodies [72]. The neutralizing antibodies are used as prophylaxis against varicella, hepatitis A, hepatitis B, rabies, and respiratory syncytial virus (RSV) infection, and they can prevent viral infection [73]. In the antiviral mAb immunotherapies, antibodies have a better activity to bind their viral targets with high affinity and specificity [74]. Hereby, mAbs block the viral entry to host cells by specifically targeting viral surface proteins, and can neutralize viral infection [75].

Considering these properties of mAbs in neutralizing other viruses, it is thought to be a therapy for COVID-19 as well. SARS-CoV-2 neutralizing mAbs recognize epitopes and prevent entrance into host cells by targeting surface S glycoproteins [73, 76], and thus they can minimize the spread of viruses and the severity of illnesses [77]. While some mAbs can prevent the interaction of RBD and ACE2 receptor by recognizing the S1 fragment of SARS-CoV, and some can recognize epitopes in the S2 unit [78].

Many studies demonstrated that SARS-CoV-2 RBD could bind to ACE2 with a similar affinity with SARS-CoV RBD [16]. Due to the similarity between SARS-CoV and SARS-CoV-2, most researchers stated that mAbs, which developed for

SARS-CoV, can also be used in SARS-CoV-2 patients [78]. Therefore, studies are carried out developing or remodified many mAbs for SARS-CoV-2 [76].

SARS-CoV-specific antibodies, m396, CR3014, and CR3022 were evaluated for their potential of binding to SARS-CoV-2 RBD. m396 and CR3014 could not bind to SARS-CoV-2 S protein, so it was showed that the difference between SARS-CoV and SARS-CoV-2 RBD has a crucial effect on the cross-reactivity of the neutralizing antibody. However, CR3022 has binding potential with RBD of SARS-CoV-2 but did not show competition for binding with ACE2 for binding, demonstrating that this antibody recognizes a different epitope that does not overlap with the ACE2 binding site. It was stated that the use of CR3022 alone or in combination with other neutralizing antibodies may have potential in the prevention and treatment of COVID-19 [16]. In the study with 14 mAbs targeting the SARS-CoV RBD, it was reported that 6 mAbs cross-reacted with SARS-CoV-2 RBD. It was informed that 7B11 and 18F3 mAbs could neutralize SARS-CoV-2 *in vitro*, and only 7B11 inhibited the binding of SARS-CoV-2 RBD to ACE2. It was also stated that although 13B6 bound strongly to SARS-CoV-2 RBD, it could not prevent SARS-CoV-2 [79]. Ejemel *et al.* stated that mAb362 was showed cross-binding activity against the RBD and S1 subunit of both the SARS-CoV-S and SARS-CoV-2-S. Both IgG and IgA isotypes of mAb362 blocked SARS-CoV-2 RBD binding to the receptor. mAb362 IgA bound to SARS-CoV-2 RBD with high affinity by competing with the ACE2 and neutralized pseudotyped SARS-CoV and SARS-CoV-2. Compared with IgG isotype, whereas IgA and IgG isotypes of mAb362 exhibited similar binding against SARS-CoV RBD, while mAb362 IgA showed better binding than IgG isotype against SARS-CoV-2 RBD. As a result, it was demonstrated that mAb362 IgA neutralized SARS-CoV-2 more potently [80].

B38, H4, and 47D11 novel mAbs have the potential to neutralize the coronavirus infection [78]. In the study with the human 47D11 antibody obtained by humanized chimeric 47D11 antibody, it was reported that the human 47D11 antibody inhibited infection of SARS-S and SARS-2-S pseudotyped [81]. In another study, the inhibition potential of whether human-origin B5, B38, H2, and H4 mAbs, isolated from a recovered patient, was showed by investigating the binding between RBD and ACE2. Results of the study showed B5 competed partially with ACE2 for RBD binding, but H2 did not compete. Contrary to this, it was found that B38 and H4 neutralized SARS-CoV-2 by blocking the binding of RBD to ACE2. Also, as the two antibodies recognize different epitopes, they have the potential to be used together. *In vivo* studies with transgenic mice indicated that H4 caused mild bronchopneumonia, but B38 did not cause any lesions [82]. Chen *et al.* indicated that human mAbs (311mAb-31B5, 311mAb-32D4, and 311mAb-31B9) which cloned from the B cell repertoire of recovered patients, bind potently and specifically to the RBD. In the study, it was reported that 311mAb-31B5 and 311mAb-32D4 antibodies blocked the interaction between SARS-CoV-2 RBD and ACE2, and inhibited SARS-CoV-2. Conversely, 311mAb-31B9 did not exhibit both blocking and neutralization activities, despite the property of bind to the RBD [75]. In another study, the isolation and efficacy of CA1 and CB6 human mAbs from a recovered patient were reported. These mAbs prevented the binding between SARS-CoV-2 RBD and ACE2, and pseudovirus transduction into Huh7, Calu-3, and HEK293T cells. While both mAbs exhibit potent neutralization activities against pseudovirus or live SARS-CoV-2 *in vitro*, CB6 shows a more potent activity than CA1. In a study in rhesus monkeys, it was also demonstrated that CB6 inhibited SARS-CoV-2, and effectively decreased viral load and ameliorated lung injury associated with infection [83]. Based on these studies, it is believed that the use of the neutralizing mAbs can effectively prevent the virus entry by targetting either RBD in S protein or a specific antibody that binds to ACE2, thus can promising to treat COVID-19 infection [84]. In a study by Liu *et al.*, 61 mAbs were isolated from 5 patients and 19 of 61 mAbs inhibited SARS-CoV-2 *in vitro*. 9 of 19 mAbs have been found to have a high neutralizing effect, and inhibited the virus, by 4 of them bind to RBD, 3 to NTD, and 2 to other epitopes. Also, *in vivo* neutralizing potency test of mAb 2-15, one of the mAbs that bind to this RBD region, has been reported to protect the hamster against SARS-CoV-2 infection [85]. In addition to these neutralizing mAbs, the efficacy of mAb drugs that previously used for different diseases is also being researched for COVID-19, as an alternative to standard therapy. One of the most investigated drugs among these mAbs is tocilizumab, known as Actemra® and RoActemra® on trade names, and was approved for rheumatoid arthritis treatment. Tocilizumab, which can block IL-6 receptors, and can prevent the inflammatory cytokine storm, by targeting excessive-induced IL-6 [86]. It is thought that tocilizumab can both inhibit signal transduction and prevent inflammatory storm by blocking IL-6 receptors in COVID-19 patients, too [87]. Also, in clinical trials with tocilizumab, it was observed that patients' fever has normalized, and respiratory function and other symptoms improved [86]. Although many researchers suggested tocilizumab is suitable for the treatment of COVID-19, they also report that clinical studies are insufficient. In a study with 544 patients with COVID-19, 179 patients received tocilizumab therapy, and 365 patients received standard therapy. In the treatment outcome, it was reported that 7% of the patients treated with tocilizumab, whereas 20% of patients treated with standard therapy died [88]. In another study, 34 of 68 patients treated with standard therapy and 7 of 90 patients treated with standard and tocilizumab therapy died. Although these results showed that the tocilizumab treatment is appropriate, the researchers stated that refers to the lack of randomization and patients in the control group was elderly with higher comorbidity prevalence [89].

In another study, 32 patients were treated with tocilizumab, and 33 patients with standard therapy until the 28th day, it was reported that 5 patients (16%) in the tocilizumab group and 11 patients (33%) in the standard therapy group died. When the patients' health status was evaluated, patients in both the tocilizumab group and standard therapy group, needed mechanical ventilation and showed severe adverse effects. This study indicates that tocilizumab treatment did not show significant improvement in patients compared to standard therapy [90]. Furthermore, Rojo *et al.* reported that tocilizumab treatment initially ameliorated the patient with COVID-19, but gastrointestinal perforation after the treatment caused the death of the patient. Intestinal perforation is one of the side effects of tocilizumab in rheumatoid arthritis treatment, may also be seen in COVID-19 treatment [91]. Even if these studies show that tocilizumab is successful and decreased mortality in the treatment of COVID-19, it has disadvantages such as side effects, outcomes that are not superior to standard therapy. In addition, tocilizumab has other side effects, including predisposition to infectious diseases such as tuberculosis, fungal, or other viral infections. As a result, more studies are needed to prove the efficiency and reliability of tocilizumab [92, 93].

LY-CoV555 (designated as Bamlanivimab) is a recombinant and fully human neutralizing IgG1 mAb, produced by Eli Lilly, has the highest binding affinity for SARS-CoV-2, and targets the RBD of the spike glycoprotein [94]. Patients received a single dose of 700, 2,800, or 7,000 mg of LY-CoV555, and the viral load change was measured at 11. day. Compared with the other groups, viral load on patients that received the 2,800 mg dose reduced, but on 700 mg and 7,000 mg doses did not significantly [95]. In addition, developed by Regeneron Pharmaceuticals, REGN-COV2 is a combination of REGN10933 (Casirivimab) and REGN10987 (Imdevimab) mAbs. These mAbs are fully human antibodies that bind to the spike protein, neutralize SARS-CoV-2, and protect against the escape of mutational virus [96]. They bind to binding domain epitopes of the nonoverlapping ACE2-competing SARS-CoV-2 receptor, inhibit virus replication, and also reduced lung pathology in Syrian hamsters and rhesus macaques [97]. REGN-COV2 has been shown effective for outpatients, and patients with mild to moderate disease, while it did not for serious patients. Therefore, these mAbs have received the Emergency Use Authorization (EUA) from the FDA, in November 2020 [95, 98].

As a conclusion, mAbs have potential in both neutralizing the infection and alleviating the disease and can be an alternative treatment approach for SARS-CoV-2. However, despite these favorable effects of mAbs, some problems limit to use of them, such as production difficulties and safety risks. Especially, the production of mAbs on a large-scale is labor-intensive, high-cost, and time-consuming. Therefore, it is a need for the production of mAbs, rapid, in a short time, and at a lower cost, particularly during an epidemic. Hence, these challenges need to be overcome, in order to be able to use mAbs on the prevention and treatment of SARS-CoV-2 infection [84].

Egg Yolk Antibodies (IgY) Against SARS-CoV-2

The immune system in chicken has some differences and it has been observed for several years. Gerrie Leslie and Bill Clem proposed in 1969 that chicken serum immunoglobulin (Ig) should be named as the egg yolk antibody (IgY) instead of IgG [99]. The reason was that the heavy (H) chains of the chicken immunoglobulin different antigenically and bigger than mammalian IgG. Because of the heavy (H) chains of the chicken immunoglobulin antigenically different than IgG and heavier than mammalian IgG. Also advancing molecular techniques have provided compelling evidence that IgY is not only the evolutionary ancestor of IgG but of IgE as well [100].

There are two heavy (H) and two light (L) chains in the structure of IgY and its molecular weight is ~180 kDa [99]. However, IgY molecular weight~120 kDa is present as a cut form in some reptiles (especially turtles), anseriform birds (ducks and geese), and lungfish [101]. Typically, heavy chains of IgY have one variable domain (V) and four constant (C) domains. Cut form of IgY lacks the two C-terminal domains in its heavy chains [102]. The isoelectric point of IgY is also lower than IgG [103].

IgY is developed by chickens to provide effective humoral immunity to their progeny against common pathogens before their immune system becomes fully mature. IgY secretion in young chicks starts 6 days after hatching [104]. After a steady serum concentration of 1.0-1.5 mg/ml, IgY secreted by mature B cells is released straight into the bloodstream [105]. Throughout the life of a chicken, the serum IgY concentration is kept constant due to the balance of the ongoing synthesis and transfer processes. Large quantities of chicken serum immunoglobulin (IgY) is transported to the embryo by egg yolk, while other Ig classes are found in negligible amounts [106]. Therefore in large amounts of IgY antibodies can be obtained from egg yolk; this enables the laying hens to become producers of high-yielding polyclonal antibodies [106]. A chicken generally lays about 280 eggs per year, and the yolk often contains 100-150 mg of IgY, showing that laying hen can produce more than 40 g of chicken antibodies (IgY) yearly [107].

Chickens can be immunized with different methods and compared to the subcutaneous injection, intramuscular injection of antigen causes the production of higher levels of antigen antibodies with approximately 10 times higher specificity [108]. Intramuscularly immunized chickens continue to produce antibodies with high specificity for more than 200 days [108]. In addition, chickens enable minimizing side effects of known immunological adjuvants such as Specol, Hunters TiterMax, Freund's adjuvant, and the lipopeptide Pam3-Cy--(lys) 4 during immunization [109].

Isolation of IgY is conducted with relatively easy precipitation methods [110] in a fluid emulsion of egg yolk consist of lipoprotein particles and lipids of egg yolk mostly exist as lipoproteins [111]. The main challenge in isolating IgY from egg yolk is separation from lipoproteins of egg yolk. The main IgY purification methods based on the removal of lipoprotein are ultracentrifugation, organic solvent delipidation, ultrafiltration, precipitation of lipoprotein, and chromatographic methods [105, 112].

IgY antibodies provide many advantages over traditional mammalian antibodies in some areas of applications. One of them is recognition of some epitopes by IgY may be better than mammalian antibodies [113]. IgY is not binding cell surface Fc receptor on mammalian cells and rheumatoid factor (RF) and does not cause human anti-mouse IgG antibodies (HAMA) reaction [114, 115]. Another advantage is the effective immune response and high antibody response is provided by less immunization compared to hybridoma methods [116]. In addition, antibody production from chickens is much less traumatic for the animal, as it is necessary to collect only eggs instead of blood [117]. The European Center for the Validation of Alternative Methods (ECVAM) also advises the use of egg yolk antibodies instead of mammalian antibodies regarding animal ethical principles [118]. One of the reasons for this recommendation is the amount of antibody corresponding to approximately 0.5 L serum taken from the animal can be obtained from a chicken within 1 month by ovulation [109]. With these advantages, IgY antibody production is more hygienic, fast, simple, cost-effective, and useful compared to obtaining antibodies from mammalian serum by traditional methods [119]. Despite the major advantages of using chickens as an antibody source over mammals, the half-life of mammalian antibodies is about 15 days, while chicken antibodies have a half-life of about 36 hours [105].

Chicken antibodies (IgY) have been used in various studies to provide effective protection and prevention against bacterial and viral infections. Oral administration of IgY has been used for the treatment of enteric infections caused by bovine-human rotaviruses, bovine coronaviruses, and enterotoxic bacteria such as *E. coli, Salmonella typhi., Edwardsiella tarda, Helicobacter pylori, ve Pseudomonas* [105, 120]. IgY is also recommended for blocking, inhibiting, and neutralizing pathogens [121]. IgYs can suppress viral colonization by preventing the spread of virus particles from cell to cell. With these features, IgYs draw attention as a promising approach for neutralizing antibody treatment against viral diseases. Studies have been conducted to neutralize some viruses that cause many different viral diseases such as Rotavirus (26), African horse sickness virus (AHSV) [122], Rabies [123], ranavirus frog virus 3 [124], Avian hepatitis E virus [125], adenovirus [126], Influenza A virus [127], Andes virus (ANDV) [128], Norovirus [129], Dengue virus [130], enterovirus and coxsackievirus [131], Zika virus [132], Canine Parvovirus [133] and Ebola [134].

Studies are also continuing against coronaviruses which are members of the Coronaviridae family and cause viral diseases that require a therapeutic and prophylactic strategy. In one of the first studies against the coronavirus family, the protective role of neutralizing anti-bovine (BCV) IgY antibodies were examined in newborn calves suffered extreme diarrhea [135]. It was observed that calves fed with egg yolk all survived while calves without any treatment (control) died within six days of infection. Results showed that egg yolk IgY antibodies administered orally protected calves against BCV infection by providing passive protection. The researchers have commented that anti-BCV IgY antibodies reacted strongly and stably in the neutralizing reaction of coronavirus epitopes *in vivo*.

In another study, neutralizing antibodies against the coronavirus and rotavirus family, anti-VP8-S IgY, was obtained by immunizing chickens with recombinant VP8-S2 protein [136]. While the coronavirus spike glycoprotein is in charge of inducing the neutralizing antibody response, the VP8 subunit of the rotavirus is the critical decisive of viral infection and neutralization. It was stated that the VP8-S2/anti-VP8-S IgY complex can be investigated as a passive vaccine candidate for coronavirus and rotavirus infections.

In the studies during the SARS epidemic in 2003, it was aimed to search for better antibody sources and increase antibody yield. In a study, it has been shown that the IgYs obtained by immunization of specific pathogen-free (SPF) chickens vaccinated with inactive SARS coronavirus, neutralized the SARS coronavirus [137]. They demonstrated that the IgY was isolated with high purity and had a good reactive behavior with a 1:640 neutralization titer by the Western blot and neutralization test. Also, stability studies showed that lyophilized anti-SARS IgY has encouraging physical characteristics, with no noticeable decrease in reactive behavior. In addition, Fu *et al.* stated that the anti-SARS IgY preparation manufactured in this research could have the potential to be commercially manufactured.

In another study in 2007, polyclonal IgY antibodies were obtained by immunized animals with recombinant SARS-CoV spike protein. Polyclonal IgY antibodies of egg yolk and serum were found to be extremely reactive to immunogenic substances when analyzed by IHC staining and Western blotting [138]. S-fragments of the *Escherichia coli* derived truncated spike protein have been shown to be an extremely good target in therapeutic and diagnostic applications.

Finally, the clinical Phase 1 study which started in September 2020 and is a clinical trial to evaluate the reliability, compatibility, and pharmacokinetics of chicken egg antibody (anti-SARS-CoV-2 IgY) against the severe acute respiratory syndrome coronavirus 2 has started (ClinicalTrials.gov Identifier: NCT04567 810). While 48 healthy participants have participated in the clinical study, the participants will be administered intranasally of anti-SARS-CoV-2 IgY in both increasing single doses and multiple doses for disease prevention. The data will be considered regarding side effects, physical assessment (including vital signs), electrocardiogram, and clinical laboratory throughput. Its pharmacokinetic properties will be evaluated by serum anti-SARS-CoV-2 IgY concentration.

On the other hand, in spite of the many benefits of IgY antibodies, applications use in investigative and medicine is restricted. One of the explanations is that the emerging problems with the immunogenicity in humans of IgY antibodies, which limits its use in the systemic implementation [139]. There are not enough reports about the systemic application and immune response of IgY antibodies in humans (Clinical Trials, 2020), and the immunogenicity of IgY in humans must be fully overcome before IgY is clinically administered.

Specific antiviral IgY has found its application in the above-mentioned studies on the coronavirus family and has shown effective results. Since therapeutic and prophylactic researches are still ongoing for the treatment of the COVID-19, it is thought that IgY may also be beneficial in therapeutic and prophylactic terms. Many prophylactic treatments, including vaccines to be developed, are in search of antibodies that have high specificity against SARS-CoV-2 and can neutralize the virus. Production of an IgY antibody takes 1.5 months from the vaccination of chickens to IgY production. Therefore, until vaccination is available for an epidemic, it eliminates an urgent medical need [140]. IgY in egg yolk produced by immunization of chickens, which is a low-cost and rapid technology for obtaining large amounts of passive immune antibodies, seems to be a very attractive option. With all these, we can say that passive immunization and neutralizing IgY antibodies against COVID-19 are promising and the application area is constantly expanding with the developing technology.

Camelid Antibodies Against SARS-CoV-2

Camelid antibodies were identified from the serum of camels by Hamers-Casterman *et al.* in 1993 as unusual antibodies that possess great antigen-binding capacities, although they lack the light chain and first constant domain (CH1)

[141]. Camelid antibodies, also called heavy-chain antibodies (HCAbs), contain only the heavy chain variable region (VH) unlike conventional antibodies comprising two variable regions (VL and VH) [142]. Even though camelid antibodies were first identified in the serum and milk of the Camelidae family such as llama, alpaca, and camel, they were later found in different species such as sharks [143].

Camelid antibodies are mainly obtained by immunizing llama, alpacas, and camels with target antigen followed by the isolation of antibodies from animal sera or milk [144, 145]. Camelid antibodies have many structural and functional advantages over conventional antibodies. The small-sized camelid antibodies provide them to reach target antigens in deep tissues much easier. Besides, camelid antibodies have high thermal and chemical stability which means that they can tolerate high temperatures, dramatic pH changes, and enzyme digestion and also they have no tendency to aggregate, therefore they can be stored for a long time without a change in their structure [142, 146]. Moreover, camelid antibodies are highly versatile, which means they can be functionalized with various modifications without losing their structural integrity [147]. However, obtaining large quantities of antibodies from camelids is a very costly and time-consuming process. As a solution, the antigen-specific fragments of camelid antibodies can be easily expressed in the laboratory and produced in large quantities using cost-effective recombinant techniques [148]. These superior features of camelid antibodies have allowed them to be involved in a variety of diagnostic and therapeutic applications and to be a promising perspective to traditional vaccine and antibody technologies [149, 150].

The heavy chain of camelid antibodies contains a variable domain called VHH that serves as the antigen-binding fragment. VHHs can also be defined as nanobodies (Nbs) or single-domain antibodies (sdAbs) due to their small size. Nanobodies have a molecular weight of 15 kDa even though HCAbs have a molecular weight of about 95 kDa, and both are much smaller than conventional antibodies (~150 kDa). Nanobodies contain high affinity and antigen-binding specificity however they have quite a short half-life [151, 152]. Besides, nanobodies are adaptable for administration through inhalation due to their favorable chemical and physical properties, making their use preferable against viral respiratory infections [153]. In addition, the short antigen-specific sequences of nanobodies can be identified from camelid serum or milk and easily expressed *in vitro* using recombinant techniques using bacteria, yeast, mammalian cells, *etc* [154].

There are various efforts to ameliorate the properties of nanobodies such as bioavailability, stability, and solubility and to integrate a new feature into their structure. The frequently used ways in the studies for engineering nanobodies are the formation of multivalent VHH constructs and VHH-fragment crystallizable (Fc) domain fusions [155]. VHH-Fc fusions, also called fusionbodies, can be generated by linking VHH to the Fc region of an IgG antibody with a hinge region, whereas multivalent constructs can be designed through a flexible amino acid sequence used to attach multiple nanobodies. Thus, the prevention of renal clearance and enhancement of the neutralization activity can be provided while various properties of nanobodies are improved [156].

The studies on the use of nanobodies as potential neutralizing agents against various diseases have been increasing over the years regarding their advantageous features [157]. One of the first studies on the application of camelid antibodies against viral infections was published in 2011 by Hultberg *et al.* In the study, heavy chain antibody fragments obtained from immunization of llamas neutralized the Respiratory Syncytial Virus (RSV), Rabies, and H5N1 Influenza viruses by specifically binding to different epitopes in the receptor-binding regions of their envelope proteins. Moreover, it was observed that the bivalent antibodies, constructed in order to increase the nanobody efficiency, had 4000 times more neutralizing potential than multivalent antibodies [158]. In recent years, it has been proven that the use of camelid antibodies as inhalable particles, and administering them to infected individuals *via* a nebulizer is an effective strategy in the treatment of respiratory infections [159]. As an example, the trivalent nanobody, ALX-0171, developed using llama antibodies by Ablynx Inc. significantly reduced the symptoms of the disease in animal models, therefore offers respirable anti-viral therapy against RSV infection [160].

It is suggested that camelid antibodies and antibody fragments have the potential to provide an effective solution against the ongoing COVID-19 pandemic, regarding their proven efficiency against other viral respiratory infections. There are already several studies in the literature in which camelid antibodies are used against MERS-CoV. In the study conducted by Zhao *et al.* in 2018, single-domain antibodies specific to MERS-CoV spike protein collected from alpacas bound to the RBD region of the spike protein and blocked the entry of the virus into host cells. The antibodies obtained from alpaca were later expressed in high amounts using *Pichia pastoris (P. pastoris)* and showed both high prophylactic and therapeutic activity in animal models created using various MERS-CoV strains [161]. Raj *et al.* developed MERS-CoV-specific nanobodies by direct cloning and expression of variable heavy chains of HCAbs which are obtained from the bone marrow of camels immunized with MERS-CoV. It was observed that these nanobodies effectively blocked MERS-CoV infection at picomolar concentrations *in vitro* by blocking the receptor-binding site of the spike protein with an exceptionally high affinity. This has demonstrated that HCAbs offer an alternative therapeutic approach for not only MERS-CoV but also other coronaviruses [162].

Studies examining the potential therapeutic application of camelid antibodies against SARS-CoV-2 have started to take place in the literature after the identification of the SARS-CoV-2 structure and the RBD of the virus [163]. Most of the researches was based on obtaining synthetic nanobodies (sybodies) using synthetic libraries without using labor-intensive and time-consuming camelid antibody production processes. For instance, Wrapp *et al.* isolated and expressed the single-domain antibody (VHH) sequences from a llama immunized with the S protein and obtained that these VHHs neutralize pseudotyped MERS-CoV and SARS-CoV viruses, and they have cross-reactivity between the spike proteins of both SARS-CoV and SARS-CoV-2. Also, these cross-reactive VHHs neutralized the SARS-CoV-2 after fused with the Fc-domain of a human IgG [14]. Consequently, this study proved that single domain antibodies can be used as useful therapeutics for SARS-CoV-2 infection. Dong *et al.* discovered the 91 lama antibodies from databases that bind to the S protein with high affinity. Later, they revealed that 15 of these antibodies prevent the binding of the ACE2 receptor with the S protein *in vivo* [164]. In their recent research, they constructed multivalent nanobodies fused to the human IgG1 Fc domain with the help of computer-aided design and obtained trivalent VHH-Fc antibodies that showed greater affinity in blocking the S1-ACE2 interaction than bivalent nanobodies in *in vitro* neutralization studies [165].

A single-domain antibody fragment named Ty1 was identified by Hanke *et al.* from alpaca that specifically binds the RBD of S protein with high specificity and affinity and blocked its interaction with ACE2. The Ty1 nanobody, which has a molecular weight of 12.8 kDa and can be expressed in large quantities in bacteria, neutralizes the SARS-CoV-2 S pseudovirus, offering a potential therapeutic antibody against SARS-CoV-2. In addition, in the study, they observed that the fusion of Ty1 to the human Fc domain greatly increased the neutralizing effect of the nanobody [166].

Li *et al.* developed 99 nanobodies by the ribosome and phage display methods using three libraries and they engineered different sorts of nanobodies to increase the effectiveness of nanobodies using several fusion techniques. One of the nanobodies, monovalent and divalent MR3 nanobody showed the highest affinity and the strongest activity for neutralizing SARS-CoV-2 pseudoviruses. Moreover, they fused MR3-MR3 with an albumin-binding domain to avoid intracellular degradation and to expand the half-life of nanobodies. They examined the *in vivo* antiviral efficacy of MR3-MR3-albumin was by infecting animals with SARS-CoV-2 and later administering a single dose of MR3-MR3-albumin nanobodies.

As a consequence, the viral load of the nanobody group was found 50 times lower than those of the control group and the divalent MR3 nanobody protected animals from SARS-CoV-2 infection and finally *in vivo* stability and the neutralization activity of nanobodies was extended owing to the functionalization [167]. Custódio *et al.* generated several sybodies that bind RBD of the S protein, in particular, sybody 23 (Sb23) displayed the highest neutralization activity against S pseudotyped viruses. They revealed that Sb23 competitively binds to the two conformations of the ACE2 binding domain on S protein by the cryo-EM analysis. Further, they confirmed that Sb23 is positioned beside the ACE2 binding domain by using the small-angle X-ray scattering (SAXS)-based modeling. As a result, they offered new epitopes available for the development of combination therapy of Sb23 with other neutralizing agents [166].

In July, a research team at Rosalind Franklin Institute discovered two neutralizing nanobodies, termed H11-D4 and H11-H4, against SARS-CoV-2 using a naive llama VHH library by phage display technique. They confirmed that these two closely related nanobodies inhibit the infection by disrupting the formation of the RBD-ACE2 complex by cryo-EM structural analysis. Finally, they constructed a chimeric nanobody by combining nanobody- human Fc domain to extend their half-life and improve affinity and specificity [168]. Gai *et al.* identified a promising therapeutic nanobody, NB11-59, derived from camel which has a significant neutralizing effect against SARS-CoV-2. NB11-59 is a small monovalent nanobody that doesn't require the Fc domain. Therefore, they produced the inhalable form of NB11-59 enables them to be easily administrated through a nebulizer on a large-scale using *P. pastoris* [169].

A study conducted by Xiang *et al.* demonstrated that different nanobody cocktails can enhance the neutralization of SARS-CoV-2. Firstly, they vaccinated a llama with RBD and then they purified single-chain antibodies that comprise high affinity and determined a substantial half-maximal inhibitory concentration (IC50) against the SARS-CoV-2 pseudotype virus. They found that nanobodies have remarkable physical and chemical stability by conducting long-term stability experiments up to 6 weeks at room temperature. Furthermore, they designed various nanobody cocktails by using the most efficient nanobody constructs such as homotrimeric nanobodies, which have one type of monovalent nanobody connected *via* a flexible linker, and heterodimeric nanobodies, which have two different monovalent nanobodies connected *via* a flexible linker. Finally, they revealed that homotrimeric constructs boosted neutralizing potency up to 30-fold relative to monovalent nanobodies while heterodimeric constructs increased up to a 4-fold in neutralization studies [153].

Schoof *et al.* explored 21 novel nanobodies that block S-ACE2 interaction by either attaching ACE2 binding site or connect elsewhere on the spike protein and indirectly hinder ACE2 binding through the allosteric regulation or the steric interference by screening yeast surface-displayed libraries. Electron microscopy analysis has shown that Nb6 and Nb11, the most potent nanobodies, interact with ACE2 binding sites competitively. To increase the binding affinity, they developed multivalent nanobodies by attaching two or three Nb6 with Gly-Ser linkers and they obtained that trivalent Nb6 nanobody occupied all three RBDs and inhibited *in vitro* SARS-CoV-2 infection. Then, they improved the neutralization activity of Nb6 approximately 200-fold higher by affinity maturation. Eventually, they performed stability studies of Nb6, mature Nb6, and trivalent Nb6 nanobodies and found that all lyophilized, heat-treated, and aerosolized nanobodies retained their stabilities and avidities, suggesting that these nanobodies can be administered intranasally [170].

Consequently, all these studies have shown that the development of camelid antibodies and antibody fragments propose a promising alternative approach for the prevention and treatment of SARS-CoV-2 infection. However, the efficiency and the reliability of the camelid antibodies and antibody fragments need further investigation.

CONCLUDING REMARKS

Since it is emerged in December 2019, the development of therapeutics and vaccines for COVID-19 has been continuing with great effort. Treatment and prevention of other coronaviruses such as SARS-CoV and MERS-CoV could be provided by the neutralizing antibodies; hence it is thought that they are also promising for neutralization of the SARS-CoV-2 virus. In this chapter, the effectiveness of antibodies was reviewed against the novel coronavirus disease, by their neutralizing effects. The studies have demonstrated that these neutralizing antibodies may be potential preventative and therapeutic agents against SARS-CoV-2, by blocking the virus entry into the host cells. Thus, it is suggested that neutralizing antibodies can prevent or treat COVID-19 by having used either alone or in combination with another. On the other hand, although the neutralizing effect of the antibodies mentioned has been shown in many different studies, more research is needed for proof of its success in COVID-19 treatment.

CONSENT FOR PUBLICATION

Not applicable.

CONFLICT OF INTEREST

The author declares no conflict of interest, financial or otherwise.

ACKNOWLEDGEMENTS

Declared none.

REFERENCES

[1]   Kannan S, Shaik Syed Ali P, Sheeza A, Hemalatha K. COVID-19 (Novel Coronavirus 2019) - recent trends. Eur Rev Med Pharmacol Sci 2020; 24(4): 2006-11.
[PMID: 32141569]

[2]   Shi Y, Wang G, Cai XP, *et al.* An overview of COVID-19. J Zhejiang Univ Sci B 2020; 21(5): 343-60.
[http://dx.doi.org/10.1631/jzus.B2000083] [PMID: 32425000]

[3]   Yuki K, Fujiogi M, Koutsogiannaki S. COVID-19 pathophysiology: A review. Clin Immunol 2020; 215: 108427.
[http://dx.doi.org/10.1016/j.clim.2020.108427] [PMID: 32325252]

[4]   Zhai P, Ding Y, Wu X, Long J, Zhong Y, Li Y. The epidemiology, diagnosis and treatment of COVID-19. Int J Antimicrob Agents 2020; 55(5): 105955.
[http://dx.doi.org/10.1016/j.ijantimicag.2020.105955] [PMID: 32234468]

[5]   Venkat Kumar G, Jeyanthi V, Ramakrishnan S. A short review on antibody therapy for COVID-19. New Microbes New Infect 2020; 35: 100682.
[http://dx.doi.org/10.1016/j.nmni.2020.100682] [PMID: 32313660]

[6]   WHO-COVID-19. Draft Landscape of COVID-19 Candidate Vaccines 2020. https://www.who.int/publications/m/item/draft-landscape-of-covid-19-candidate-vaccines

[7]   Oliver SE, Gargano JW, Marin M, *et al.* The Advisory Committee on Immunization Practices' Interim Recommendation for Use of Pfizer-BioNTech COVID-19 Vaccine - United States, December 2020. MMWR Morb Mortal Wkly Rep 2020; 69(50): 1922-4.
[http://dx.doi.org/10.15585/mmwr.mm6950e2] [PMID: 33332292]

[8]   Oliver SE, Gargano JW, Marin M, *et al.* The Advisory Committee on Immunization Practices' Interim Recommendation for Use of Moderna COVID-19 Vaccine - United States, December 2020. MMWR Morb Mortal Wkly Rep 2021; 69(5152): 1653-6.
[http://dx.doi.org/10.15585/mmwr.mm695152e1] [PMID: 33382675]

[9]   Ramasamy MN, Minassian AM, Ewer KJ, *et al.* Safety and immunogenicity of ChAdOx1 nCoV-19 vaccine administered in a prime-boost regimen in young and old adults (COV002): a single-blind, randomised, controlled, phase 2/3 trial. Lancet 2021; 396(10267): 1979-93.
[http://dx.doi.org/10.1016/S0140-6736(20)32466-1] [PMID: 33220855]

[10]   Plotkin SA. Vaccines: past, present and future. Nat Med 2005; 11(4) (Suppl.): S5-S11.
[http://dx.doi.org/10.1038/nm1209] [PMID: 15812490]

[11]   Plotkin SA. Vaccines: the fourth century. Clin Vaccine Immunol 2009; 16(12): 1709-19.
[http://dx.doi.org/10.1128/CVI.00290-09] [PMID: 19793898]

[12]   Ku Z, Ye X. Salazar GTa, Zhang N, An Z. Antibody therapies for the treatment of COVID-19. Antibody Therapeutics 2020; 3(2): 101-8.
[http://dx.doi.org/10.1093/abt/tbaa007]

[13]   Wrapp D, Wang N, Corbett KS, *et al.* Cryo-EM structure of the 2019-nCoV spike in the prefusion conformation. Science 2020; 367(6483): 1260-3.

[http://dx.doi.org/10.1126/science.abb2507] [PMID: 32075877]

[14]   Wrapp D, De Vlieger D, Corbett KS, *et al.* Structural Basis for Potent Neutralization of Betacoronaviruses by Single-Domain Camelid Antibodies. Cell 2020; 181(5): 1004-1015.e15.
[http://dx.doi.org/10.1016/j.cell.2020.04.031] [PMID: 32375025]

[15]   Ahn DG, Shin HJ, Kim MH, *et al.* Current Status of Epidemiology, Diagnosis, Therapeutics, and Vaccines for Novel Coronavirus Disease 2019 (COVID-19). J Microbiol Biotechnol 2020; 30(3): 313-24.
[http://dx.doi.org/10.4014/jmb.2003.03011] [PMID: 32238757]

[16]   Tian X, Li C, Huang A, *et al.* Potent binding of 2019 novel coronavirus spike protein by a SARS coronavirus-specific human monoclonal antibody. Emerg Microbes Infect 2020; 9(1): 382-5.
[http://dx.doi.org/10.1080/22221751.2020.1729069] [PMID: 32065055]

[17]   Koeppen BM, Stanton BA. Berne & Levy Physiology. Updated Edition E-Book: Elsevier Health Sciences 2009.

[18]   Marano G, Vaglio S, Pupella S, *et al.* Convalescent plasma: new evidence for an old therapeutic tool? Blood Transfus 2016; 14(2): 152-7.
[PMID: 26674811]

[19]   Shahani L, Singh S, Khardori NM. Immunotherapy in clinical medicine: historical perspective and current status. Med Clin North Am 2012; 96(3): 421-431, ix.
[http://dx.doi.org/10.1016/j.mcna.2012.04.001] [PMID: 22703849]

[20]   Shakir EM, Cheung DS, Grayson MH. Mechanisms of immunotherapy: a historical perspective. Ann Allergy Asthma Immunol 2010; 105(5): 340-7.
[http://dx.doi.org/10.1016/j.anai.2010.09.012] [PMID: 21055659]

[21]   Hess AF. A protective therapy for mumps. Am J Dis Child 1915; 10(2): 99-103.

[22]   Marson P, Cozza A, De Silvestro G. The true historical origin of convalescent plasma therapy. Transfusion and apheresis science : official journal of the World Apheresis Association : official journal of the European Society for Haemapheresis 2020; 102847.

[23]   Pontecorvo M. Storia delle vaccinazioni: dalle origini ai nostri giorni: Ciba-Geigy Edizioni; 1991

[24]   Flicker S, Linhart B, Wild C, Wiedermann U, Valenta R. Passive immunization with allergen-specific IgG antibodies for treatment and prevention of allergy. Immunobiology 2013; 218(6): 884-91.
[http://dx.doi.org/10.1016/j.imbio.2012.10.008] [PMID: 23182706]

[25]   Lachmann PJ. The use of antibodies in the prophylaxis and treatment of infections. Emerg Microbes Infect 2012; 1(8): e11.
[http://dx.doi.org/10.1038/emi.2012.2] [PMID: 26038423]

[26]   Stangel M, Pul R. Basic principles of intravenous immunoglobulin (IVIg) treatment. J Neurol 2006; 253(5) (Suppl. 5): V18-24.
[http://dx.doi.org/10.1007/s00415-006-5003-1] [PMID: 16998749]

[27]   Rojas M, Rodríguez Y, Monsalve DM, *et al.* Convalescent plasma in Covid-19: Possible mechanisms of action. Autoimmun Rev 2020; 19(7): 102554.
[http://dx.doi.org/10.1016/j.autrev.2020.102554] [PMID: 32380316]

[28]   Soo YOY, Cheng Y, Wong R, *et al.* Retrospective comparison of convalescent plasma with continuing high-dose methylprednisolone treatment in SARS patients. Clin Microbiol Infect 2004; 10(7): 676-8.
[http://dx.doi.org/10.1111/j.1469-0691.2004.00956.x] [PMID: 15214887]

[29]   Cheng Y, Wong R, Soo YOY, *et al.* Use of convalescent plasma therapy in SARS patients in Hong Kong. Eur J Clin Microbiol Infect Dis 2005; 24(1): 44-6.
[http://dx.doi.org/10.1007/s10096-004-1271-9] [PMID: 15616839]

[30]   Yeh K-M, Chiueh T-S, Siu LK, *et al.* Experience of using convalescent plasma for severe acute respiratory syndrome among healthcare workers in a Taiwan hospital. J Antimicrob Chemother 2005;

56(5): 919-22.
[http://dx.doi.org/10.1093/jac/dki346] [PMID: 16183666]

[31]   Ko J-H, Seok H, Cho SY, *et al.* Challenges of convalescent plasma infusion therapy in Middle East respiratory coronavirus infection: a single centre experience. Antivir Ther 2018; 23(7): 617-22.
[http://dx.doi.org/10.3851/IMP3243] [PMID: 29923831]

[32]   Chen L, Xiong J, Bao L, Shi Y. Convalescent plasma as a potential therapy for COVID-19. Lancet Infect Dis 2020; 20(4): 398-400.
[http://dx.doi.org/10.1016/S1473-3099(20)30141-9] [PMID: 32113510]

[33]   Rajendran K, Krishnasamy N, Rangarajan J, Rathinam J, Natarajan M, Ramachandran A. Convalescent plasma transfusion for the treatment of COVID-19: Systematic review. J Med Virol 2020; 92(9): 1475-83.
[http://dx.doi.org/10.1002/jmv.25961] [PMID: 32356910]

[34]   Shen C, Wang Z, Zhao F, *et al.* Treatment of 5 critically ill patients with COVID-19 with convalescent plasma. JAMA 2020; 323(16): 1582-9.
[http://dx.doi.org/10.1001/jama.2020.4783] [PMID: 32219428]

[35]   Huaxia. China puts 245 COVID-19 patients on convalescent plasma therapy. http://www.xinhuanet.com/english/2020-02/28/c_138828177.htm2020

[36]   Duan K, Liu B, Li C, *et al.* Effectiveness of convalescent plasma therapy in severe COVID-19 patients. Proc Natl Acad Sci USA 2020; 117(17): 9490-6.
[http://dx.doi.org/10.1073/pnas.2004168117] [PMID: 32253318]

[37]   Ye M, Fu D, Ren Y, *et al.* Treatment with convalescent plasma for COVID-19 patients in Wuhan, China. J Med Virol 2020; 92(10): 1890-901.
[http://dx.doi.org/10.1002/jmv.25882] [PMID: 32293713]

[38]   Salazar E, Christensen PA, Graviss EA, *et al.* Treatment of coronavirus disease 2019 patients with convalescent plasma reveals a signal of significantly decreased mortality. Am J Pathol 2020; 190(11): 2290-303.
[http://dx.doi.org/10.1016/j.ajpath.2020.08.001] [PMID: 32795424]

[39]   Hegerova L, Gooley TA, Sweerus KA, *et al.* Use of convalescent plasma in hospitalized patients with COVID-19: case series. Blood 2020; 136(6): 759-62.
[http://dx.doi.org/10.1182/blood.2020006964] [PMID: 32559767]

[40]   Liu STH, Lin H-M, Baine I, *et al.* Convalescent plasma treatment of severe COVID-19: a propensity score-matched control study. Nat Med 2020; 26(11): 1708-13.
[http://dx.doi.org/10.1038/s41591-020-1088-9] [PMID: 32934372]

[41]   Abolghasemi H, Eshghi P, Cheraghali AM, *et al.* Clinical efficacy of convalescent plasma for treatment of COVID-19 infections: Results of a multicenter clinical study. Transfus Apheresis Sci 2020; 59(5): 102875.
[http://dx.doi.org/10.1016/j.transci.2020.102875] [PMID: 32694043]

[42]   Li L, Zhang W, Hu Y, *et al.* Effect of Convalescent Plasma Therapy on Time to Clinical Improvement in Patients With Severe and Life-threatening COVID-19: A Randomized Clinical Trial. JAMA 2020; 324(5): 460-70.
[http://dx.doi.org/10.1001/jama.2020.10044] [PMID: 32492084]

[43]   Liu J, Li S, Liu J, *et al.* Longitudinal characteristics of lymphocyte responses and cytokine profiles in the peripheral blood of SARS-CoV-2 infected patients. EBioMedicine 2020; 55: 102763.
[http://dx.doi.org/10.1016/j.ebiom.2020.102763] [PMID: 32361250]

[44]   Zhao J, Yuan Q, Wang H, *et al.* Antibody responses to SARS-CoV-2 in patients of novel coronavirus disease 2019. Clin Infect Dis 2020; 71(16): 2027-34.
[http://dx.doi.org/10.1093/cid/ciaa344] [PMID: 32221519]

[45]   Amanat F, Stadlbauer D, Strohmeier S, *et al.* A serological assay to detect SARS-CoV-2

seroconversion in humans. Nat Med 2020; 26(7): 1033-6.
[http://dx.doi.org/10.1038/s41591-020-0913-5] [PMID: 32398876]

[46]   Research USDoHaHSFaDACfBEa. Investigational COVID-19 convalescent plasma - guidance for industry. 2020.

[47]   Yiğenoğlu TN, Hacıbekiroğlu T, Berber İ, *et al.* Convalescent plasma therapy in patients with COVID-19. J Clin Apher 2020; 35(4): 367-73.
[http://dx.doi.org/10.1002/jca.21806] [PMID: 32643200]

[48]   Safety EC-D-GfHaF. An EU programme of COVID-19 convalescent plasma collection and transfusion: guidance on collection, testing, processing, storage, distribution and monitored use. Brussels, Belgium 2020.

[49]   Liu W, Fontanet A, Zhang P-H, *et al.* Two-year prospective study of the humoral immune response of patients with severe acute respiratory syndrome. J Infect Dis 2006; 193(6): 792-5.
[http://dx.doi.org/10.1086/500469] [PMID: 16479513]

[50]   Jaume M, Yip MS, Cheung CY, *et al.* Anti-severe acute respiratory syndrome coronavirus spike antibodies trigger infection of human immune cells *via* a pH- and cysteine protease-independent FcγR pathway. J Virol 2011; 85(20): 10582-97.
[http://dx.doi.org/10.1128/JVI.00671-11] [PMID: 21775467]

[51]   Sharun K, Tiwari R, Iqbal Yatoo M, *et al.* Antibody-based immunotherapeutics and use of convalescent plasma to counter COVID-19: advances and prospects. Expert Opin Biol Ther 2020; 20(9): 1033-46.
[http://dx.doi.org/10.1080/14712598.2020.1796963] [PMID: 32744917]

[52]   Joyner M, Wright RS, Fairweather D, *et al.* Early safety indicators of COVID-19 convalescent plasma in 5,000 patients. medRxiv 2020; 2020.05.12.20099879.
[PMID: 32511566]

[53]   Joyner MJ, Bruno KA, Klassen SA, Kunze KL, Johnson PW, Lesser ER, Eds. Safety update: COVID-19 convalescent plasma in 20,000 hospitalized patients. Elsevier 2020.
[http://dx.doi.org/10.1016/j.mayocp.2020.06.028]

[54]   Khadka S, Saleem M, Shrestha D, Budhathoki P. Safety and efficacy of convalescent plasma therapy for the management of COVID-19. Syst Rev 2020.

[55]   Mair-Jenkins J, Saavedra-Campos M, Baillie JK, *et al.* Convalescent Plasma Study Group. The effectiveness of convalescent plasma and hyperimmune immunoglobulin for the treatment of severe acute respiratory infections of viral etiology: a systematic review and exploratory meta-analysis. J Infect Dis 2015; 211(1): 80-90.
[http://dx.doi.org/10.1093/infdis/jiu396] [PMID: 25030060]

[56]   Köhler G, Milstein CJn. Continuous cultures of fused cells secreting antibody of predefined specificity. 1975; 256(5517): 495-7.

[57]   Pandey SJH. Hybridoma technology for production of monoclonal antibodies 2010; 1(2): 017.

[58]   Knapp FR, Dash A. Radioimmunotherapy (RIT) Radiopharmaceuticals for Therapy. Springer 2016; pp. 169-84.
[http://dx.doi.org/10.1007/978-81-322-2607-9_9]

[59]   Bonnevier J, Hammerbeck C, Goetz C. Flow Cytometry: Definition, History, and Uses in Biological Research Flow Cytometry Basics for the Non-Expert. Springer 2018; pp. 1-11.

[60]   Gad SC. Drug safety evaluation. John Wiley & Sons 2016.
[http://dx.doi.org/10.1002/9781119097440]

[61]   Jin Y, Lei C, Hu D, Dimitrov DS, TJFom Ying. Human monoclonal antibodies as candidate therapeutics against emerging viruses. 2017; 11(4): 462-70.

[62]   Sodoyer RJBoMA. The history of therapeutic monoclonal antibodies. 2016; 1-62.

[63] Lynch C, Grewal I. Preclinical safety evaluation of monoclonal antibodies Therapeutic Antibodies. Springer 2008; pp. 19-44.

[64] Lonberg NJCoii. Fully human antibodies from transgenic mouse and phage display platforms. 2008; 20(4): 450-9.

[65] Sheets MD, Amersdorfer P, Finnern R, Sargent P, Lindqvist E, Schier R, *et al.* Efficient construction of a large nonimmune phage antibody library: the production of high-affinity human single-chain antibodies to protein antigens. 1998; 95(11): 6157-2.
[http://dx.doi.org/10.1073/pnas.95.11.6157]

[66] Liu B, Huang L, Sihlböm C, Burlingame A, Marks JDJJomb. Towards proteome-wide production of monoclonal antibody by phage display. 2002; 315(5): 1063-73.

[67] Murphy AJ, Macdonald LE, Stevens S, Karow M, Dore AT, Pobursky K, *et al.* Mice with megabase humanization of their immunoglobulin genes generate antibodies as efficiently as normal mice. 2014; 111(14): 5153-8.
[http://dx.doi.org/10.1073/pnas.1324022111]

[68] Sok D, Briney B, Jardine JG, Kulp DW, Menis S, Pauthner M, *et al.* Priming HIV-1 broadly neutralizing antibody precursors in human Ig loci transgenic mice. 2016; 353(6307): 1557-60.
[http://dx.doi.org/10.1126/science.aah3945]

[69] Nissim A, Chernajovsky Y. Historical development of monoclonal antibody therapeutics Therapeutic Antibodies. Springer 2008; pp. 3-18.

[70] Anand B, Deng R, Theil F-P, Li J, Jumbe S, Gelzleichter T, *et al.* Monoclonal Antibodies: From Structure to Therapeutic Applications Pharmaceutical Biotechnology. CRC Press 2016; pp. 325-54.

[71] Scott LJ, Lamb HMJD. Palivizumab 1999; 58(2): 305-11.

[72] Du L, Zhao G, Yang Y, Qiu H, Wang L, Kou Z, *et al.* A conformation-dependent neutralizing monoclonal antibody specifically targeting receptor-binding domain in Middle East respiratory syndrome coronavirus spike protein. 2014; 88(12): 7045-53.
[http://dx.doi.org/10.1128/JVI.00433-14]

[73] Greenough TC, Babcock GJ, Roberts A, Hernandez HJ, Thomas WD Jr, Coccia JA, *et al.* Development and characterization of a severe acute respiratory syndrome—associated coronavirus—neutralizing human monoclonal antibody that provides effective immunoprophylaxis in mice. 2005; 191(4): 507-14.

[74] Marasco WA. Sui JJNb.. The growth and potential of human antiviral monoclonal antibody therapeutics. 2007; 25(12): 1421-34.

[75] Chen X, Li R, Pan Z, Qian C, Yang Y, You R, *et al.* Human monoclonal antibodies block the binding of SARS-CoV-2 spike protein to angiotensin converting enzyme 2 receptor. 2020; 1-3.
[http://dx.doi.org/10.1038/s41423-020-0426-7]

[76] Marovich M, Mascola JR, Cohen MSJJ. Monoclonal antibodies for prevention and treatment of COVID-19. 2020; 324(2): 131-2.

[77] Walker LM, Burton DRJNRI. Passive immunotherapy of viral infections:'super-antibodies' enter the fray. 2018; 18(5): 297.

[78] Jahanshahlu L, Rezaei NJB. Pharmacotherapy. Monoclonal Antibody as a Potential Anti-COVID 2020; 19: 110337.

[79] Tai W, Zhang X, He Y, Jiang S, Du LJAR. Identification of SARS-CoV RBD-targeting monoclonal antibodies with cross-reactive or neutralizing activity against SARS-CoV-2. 2020; 104820.

[80] Ejemel M, Li Q, Hou S, Schiller ZA, Tree JA, Wallace A, *et al.* A cross-reactive human IgA monoclonal antibody blocks SARS-CoV-2 spike-ACE2 interaction. 2020; 11(1): 1-9.

[81] Wang C, Li W, Drabek D, Okba NM, van Haperen R, Osterhaus AD, *et al.* A human monoclonal

antibody blocking SARS-CoV-2 infection. 2020; 11(1): 1-6.

[82]   Wu Y, Wang F, Shen C, Peng W, Li D, Zhao C, *et al.* A noncompeting pair of human neutralizing antibodies block COVID-19 virus binding to its receptor ACE2. 2020; 368(6496): 1274-8.
[http://dx.doi.org/10.1126/science.abc2241]

[83]   Shi R, Shan C, Duan X, Chen Z, Liu P, Song J, *et al.* A human neutralizing antibody targets the receptor binding site of SARS-CoV-2. 2020; 1-8.
[http://dx.doi.org/10.1038/s41586-020-2381-y]

[84]   Shanmugaraj B, Siriwattananon K, Wangkanont K, Phoolcharoen WJAPJAI. Perspectives on monoclonal antibody therapy as potential therapeutic intervention for Coronavirus disease-19 (COVID-19). 2020; 38(1): 10-8.

[85]   Liu L, Wang P, Nair MS, *et al.* Potent neutralizing antibodies against multiple epitopes on SARS-CoV-2 spike. Nature 2020; 584(7821): 450-6.
[http://dx.doi.org/10.1038/s41586-020-2571-7] [PMID: 32698192]

[86]   Fu B, Xu X. Wei HJJotm.. Why tocilizumab could be an effective treatment for severe COVID-19? 2020; 18(1): 1-5.

[87]   Zhang S, Li L, Shen A, Chen Y, Qi ZJCDI. Rational use of tocilizumab in the treatment of novel coronavirus pneumonia. 2020; 40(6): 511-8.
[http://dx.doi.org/10.1007/s40261-020-00917-3]

[88]   Schulert GSJTLR. Can tocilizumab calm the cytokine storm of COVID-19? 2020; 2(8): e449-51.

[89]   De Rossi N, Scarpazza C, Filippini C, Cordioli C, Rasia S, Mancinelli CR, *et al.* Early use of low dose tocilizumab in patients with COVID-19: A retrospective cohort study with a complete follow-up. 2020; 25: 100459.

[90]   Campochiaro C, Della-Torre E, Cavalli G, De Luca G, Ripa M, Boffini N, *et al.* Efficacy and safety of tocilizumab in severe COVID-19 patients: a single-centre retrospective cohort study. 2020.
[http://dx.doi.org/10.1016/j.ejim.2020.05.021]

[91]   Rojo M, Cano-Valderrama O, Picazo S, Saez C, Gómez L, Sánchez C, *et al.* Gastrointestinal perforation after treatment with tocilizumab: an unexpected consequence of COVID-19 pandemic. 2020; 86(6): 565-6.

[92]   Zhao MJIjoaa. Cytokine storm and immunomodulatory therapy in COVID-19: role of chloroquine and anti-IL-6 monoclonal antibodies. 2020.

[93]   Zhang Y, Zhong Y, Pan L, Dong JJDD. Therapeutics. Treat 2019 novel coronavirus (COVID-19) with IL-6 inhibitor: Are we already that far? 2020; 14(2): 100-2.

[94]   Tuccori M, Ferraro S, Convertino I, *et al.* Anti-SARS-CoV-2 neutralizing monoclonal antibodies: clinical pipeline. MAbs 2020; 12(1): 1854149.
[http://dx.doi.org/10.1080/19420862.2020.1854149] [PMID: 33319649]

[95]   Jiang S, Zhang X, Yang Y, Hotez PJ, Du L. Neutralizing antibodies for the treatment of COVID-19. Nat Biomed Eng 2020; 4(12): 1134-9.
[http://dx.doi.org/10.1038/s41551-020-00660-2] [PMID: 33293725]

[96]   Baum A, Ajithdoss D, Copin R, *et al.* REGN-COV2 antibodies prevent and treat SARS-CoV-2 infection in rhesus macaques and hamsters. Science 2020; 370(6520): 1110-5.
[http://dx.doi.org/10.1126/science.abe2402] [PMID: 33037066]

[97]   Shafer RW A. A SARS-CoV-2 antiviral therapy score card. Global Health & Medicine 2020.

[98]   Pardi N, Weissman D. Development of vaccines and antivirals for combating viral pandemics. Nat Biomed Eng 2020; 4(12): 1128-33.
[http://dx.doi.org/10.1038/s41551-020-00658-w] [PMID: 33293724]

[99]   Leslie GA, Clem LW. Phylogen of immunoglobulin structure and function. 3. Immunoglobulins of the

chicken. J Exp Med 1969; 130(6): 1337-52.
[http://dx.doi.org/10.1084/jem.130.6.1337] [PMID: 5352783]

[100] Warr GW, Magor KE, Higgins DA. IgY: clues to the origins of modern antibodies. Immunol Today 1995; 16(8): 392-8.
[http://dx.doi.org/10.1016/0167-5699(95)80008-5] [PMID: 7546196]

[101] Amemiya CT, Haire RN, Litman GW. Nucleotide sequence of a cDNA encoding a third distinct Xenopus immunoglobulin heavy chain isotype. Nucleic Acids Res 1989; 17(13): 5388.
[http://dx.doi.org/10.1093/nar/17.13.5388] [PMID: 2503814]

[102] Fellah JS, Kerfourn F, Wiles MV, Schwager J, Charlemagne J. Phylogeny of immunoglobulin heavy chain isotypes: structure of the constant region of Ambystoma mexicanum upsilon chain deduced from cDNA sequence. Immunogenetics 1993; 38(5): 311-7.
[http://dx.doi.org/10.1007/BF00210471] [PMID: 8344718]

[103] Polson A, von Wechmar MB, Fazakerley G. Antibodies to proteins from yolk of immunized hens. Immunol Commun 1980; 9(5): 495-514.
[http://dx.doi.org/10.3109/08820138009066011] [PMID: 6776029]

[104] Davies EL, Smith JS, Birkett CR, Manser JM, Anderson-Dear DV, Young JR. Selection of specific phage-display antibodies using libraries derived from chicken immunoglobulin genes. J Immunol Methods 1995; 186(1): 125-35.
[http://dx.doi.org/10.1016/0022-1759(95)00143-X] [PMID: 7561141]

[105] Dias da Silva W, Tambourgi DV. IgY: a promising antibody for use in immunodiagnostic and in immunotherapy. Vet Immunol Immunopathol 2010; 135(3-4): 173-80.
[http://dx.doi.org/10.1016/j.vetimm.2009.12.011] [PMID: 20083313]

[106] Carlander D, Stålberg J, Larsson A. Chicken antibodies: a clinical chemistry perspective. Ups J Med Sci 1999; 104(3): 179-89.
[http://dx.doi.org/10.3109/03009739909178961] [PMID: 10680951]

[107] Mine Y, Kovacs-Nolan J. Chicken egg yolk antibodies as therapeutics in enteric infectious disease: a review. J Med Food 2002; 5(3): 159-69.
[http://dx.doi.org/10.1089/10966200260398198] [PMID: 12495588]

[108] Woolley JA, Landon J. Comparison of antibody production to human interleukin-6 (IL-6) by sheep and chickens. J Immunol Methods 1995; 178(2): 253-65.
[http://dx.doi.org/10.1016/0022-1759(94)00263-V] [PMID: 7836787]

[109] Lösch U, Schranner I, Wanke R, Jürgens L. The chicken egg, an antibody source. Zentralblatt fur Veterinarmedizin Reihe B Journal of veterinary medicine Series B 1986; 33(8): 609-19.
[http://dx.doi.org/10.1111/j.1439-0450.1986.tb00076.x]

[110] Bizanov G. IgY extraction and purification from chicken egg yolk. J Hell Vet Med Soc 2018; 68: 265.
[http://dx.doi.org/10.12681/jhvms.15466]

[111] Horikoshi T, Hiraoka J, Saito M, Hamada S. IgG Antibody from Hen Egg Yolks: Purification by Ethanol Fractionation. J Food Sci 2006; 58: 739-42.
[http://dx.doi.org/10.1111/j.1365-2621.1993.tb09348.x]

[112] Schade R, Calzado EG, Sarmiento R, Chacana PA, Porankiewicz-Asplund J, Terzolo HR. Chicken egg yolk antibodies (IgY-technology): a review of progress in production and use in research and human and veterinary medicine. Altern Lab Anim 2005; 33(2): 129-54.
[http://dx.doi.org/10.1177/026119290503300208] [PMID: 16180988]

[113] Song CS, Yu JH, Bai DH, Hester PY, Kim KH. Antibodies to the alpha-subunit of insulin receptor from eggs of immunized hens. J Immunol 1985; 135(5): 3354-9.
[PMID: 4045194]

[114] Gardner PS, Kaye S. Egg globulins in rapid virus diagnosis. J Virol Methods 1982; 4(4-5): 257-62.
[http://dx.doi.org/10.1016/0166-0934(82)90072-6] [PMID: 6286706]

[115] Larsson A, Karlsson-Parra A, Sjöquist J. Use of chicken antibodies in enzyme immunoassays to avoid interference by rheumatoid factors. Clin Chem 1991; 37(3): 411-4.
[http://dx.doi.org/10.1093/clinchem/37.3.411] [PMID: 2004449]

[116] Larsson A, Carlander D, Wilhelmsson M. Antibody response in laying hens with small amounts of antigen. Food Agric Immunol 1998; 10(1): 29-36.
[http://dx.doi.org/10.1080/09540109809354966]

[117] Schade R, Pfister C, Halatsch R. Henklein PJAtLA.. Polyclonal IgY antibodies from chicken egg yolk—an alternative to the production of mammalian IgG type antibodies in rabbits. 1991; 19(4): 403-19.

[118] Carlander D, Kollberg H, Wejåker PE, Larsson A. Peroral immunotherapy with yolk antibodies for the prevention and treatment of enteric infections. Immunol Res 2000; 21(1): 1-6.
[http://dx.doi.org/10.1385/IR:21:1:1] [PMID: 10803878]

[119] Zhang WW. The use of gene-specific IgY antibodies for drug target discovery. Drug Discov Today 2003; 8(8): 364-71.
[http://dx.doi.org/10.1016/S1359-6446(03)02655-2] [PMID: 12681940]

[120] Kuroki M, Ikemori Y, Yokoyama H, Peralta RC, Icatlo FC Jr, Kodama Y. Passive protection against bovine rotavirus-induced diarrhea in murine model by specific immunoglobulins from chicken egg yolk. Vet Microbiol 1993; 37(1-2): 135-46.
[http://dx.doi.org/10.1016/0378-1135(93)90188-D] [PMID: 8296443]

[121] Spillner E, Braren I, Greunke K, Seismann H, Blank S, du Plessis D. Avian IgY antibodies and their recombinant equivalents in research, diagnostics and therapy. Biologicals 2012; 40(5): 313-22.
[http://dx.doi.org/10.1016/j.biologicals.2012.05.003] [PMID: 22748514]

[122] Bentley L, Fehrsen J, Jordaan F, Huismans H, du Plessis DH. Identification of antigenic regions on VP2 of African horsesickness virus serotype 3 by using phage-displayed epitope libraries. J Gen Virol 2000; 81(Pt 4): 993-1000.
[http://dx.doi.org/10.1099/0022-1317-81-4-993] [PMID: 10725425]

[123] Motoi Y, Sato K, Hatta H, Morimoto K, Inoue S, Yamada A. Production of rabies neutralizing antibody in hen's eggs using a part of the G protein expressed in Escherichia coli. Vaccine 2005; 23(23): 3026-32.
[http://dx.doi.org/10.1016/j.vaccine.2004.11.071] [PMID: 15811649]

[124] Maniero GD, Morales H, Gantress J, Robert J. Generation of a long-lasting, protective, and neutralizing antibody response to the ranavirus FV3 by the frog Xenopus. Dev Comp Immunol 2006; 30(7): 649-57.
[http://dx.doi.org/10.1016/j.dci.2005.09.007] [PMID: 16380162]

[125] Guo H, Zhou EM, Sun ZF, Meng XJ. Immunodominant epitopes mapped by synthetic peptides on the capsid protein of avian hepatitis E virus are non-protective. Viral Immunol 2008; 21(1): 61-7.
[http://dx.doi.org/10.1089/vim.2007.0082] [PMID: 18355123]

[126] Greenall SA, Tyack SG, Johnson MA, Sapats SI. Antibody fragments, expressed by a fowl adenovirus vector, are able to neutralize infectious bursal disease virus. Avian Pathol 2010; 39(5): 339-48.
[http://dx.doi.org/10.1080/03079457.2010.507239] [PMID: 20954010]

[127] Thangavel RR, Reed A, Norcross EW, Dixon SN, Marquart ME, Stray SJ. "Boom" and "Bust" cycles in virus growth suggest multiple selective forces in influenza a evolution. Virol J 2011; 8(1): 180.
[http://dx.doi.org/10.1186/1743-422X-8-180] [PMID: 21501520]

[128] Brocato R, Josleyn M, Ballantyne J, Vial P, Hooper JW. DNA vaccine-generated duck polyclonal antibodies as a postexposure prophylactic to prevent hantavirus pulmonary syndrome (HPS). PLoS One 2012; 7(4): e35996.
[http://dx.doi.org/10.1371/journal.pone.0035996] [PMID: 22558299]

[129] Dai Y-C, Wang Y-Y, Zhang X-F, *et al.* Evaluation of anti-norovirus IgY from egg yolk of chickens

immunized with norovirus P particles. J Virol Methods 2012; 186(1-2): 126-31.
[http://dx.doi.org/10.1016/j.jviromet.2012.07.002] [PMID: 22867844]

[130] Fink AL, Williams KL, Harris E, *et al.* Dengue virus specific IgY provides protection following lethal dengue virus challenge and is neutralizing in the absence of inducing antibody dependent enhancement. PLoS Negl Trop Dis 2017; 11(7): e0005721.
[http://dx.doi.org/10.1371/journal.pntd.0005721] [PMID: 28686617]

[131] Gao E, Wu S, Xu Q, *et al.* Enterovirus type 71-immunized chicken egg yolk immunoglobulin has cross antiviral activity against coxsackievirus A16 *in vitro.* Exp Ther Med 2019; 18(1): 332-41.
[http://dx.doi.org/10.3892/etm.2019.7529] [PMID: 31258670]

[132] O'Donnell KL, Meberg B, Schiltz J, Nilles ML, Bradley DS. Zika Virus-Specific IgY Results Are Therapeutic Following a Lethal Zika Virus Challenge without Inducing Antibody-Dependent Enhancement. Viruses 2019; 11(3): 301.
[http://dx.doi.org/10.3390/v11030301] [PMID: 30917523]

[133] Ge S, Xu L, Li B, Zhong F, Liu X, Zhang X. Canine Parvovirus is diagnosed and neutralized by chicken IgY-scFv generated against the virus capsid protein. Vet Res (Faisalabad) 2020; 51(1): 110.
[http://dx.doi.org/10.1186/s13567-020-00832-7] [PMID: 32883344]

[134] Pérez de la Lastra JM, Baca-González V, Asensio-Calavia P, González-Acosta S, Morales-delaNuez A. Can immunization of hens provide oral-based therapeutics against COVID-19? Vaccines (Basel) 2020; 8(3): 486.
[http://dx.doi.org/10.3390/vaccines8030486] [PMID: 32872186]

[135] Ikemori Y, Ohta M, Umeda K, *et al.* Passive protection of neonatal calves against bovine coronavirus-induced diarrhea by administration of egg yolk or colostrum antibody powder. Vet Microbiol 1997; 58(2-4): 105-11.
[http://dx.doi.org/10.1016/S0378-1135(97)00144-2] [PMID: 9453122]

[136] Nasiri K, Nassiri MR, Tahmoorespur M, Haghparast A, Zibaee S. Production and characterization of egg yolk antibody (IgY) against recombinant VP8-S2 antigen. Pol J Vet Sci 2016; 19(2): 271-9.
[http://dx.doi.org/10.1515/pjvs-2016-0034] [PMID: 27487500]

[137] Fu C-Y, Huang H, Wang X-M, *et al.* Preparation and evaluation of anti-SARS coronavirus IgY from yolks of immunized SPF chickens. J Virol Methods 2006; 133(1): 112-5.
[http://dx.doi.org/10.1016/j.jviromet.2005.10.027] [PMID: 16325277]

[138] Lee Y-C, Leu S-JC, Hung H-C, *et al.* A dominant antigenic epitope on SARS-CoV spike protein identified by an avian single-chain variable fragment (scFv)-expressing phage. Vet Immunol Immunopathol 2007; 117(1-2): 75-85.
[http://dx.doi.org/10.1016/j.vetimm.2007.02.001] [PMID: 17360045]

[139] Xiao Y, Gao X. Use of IgY antibodies and semiconductor nanocrystal detection in cancer biomarker quantitation. Biomarkers Med 2010; 4(2): 227-39.
[http://dx.doi.org/10.2217/bmm.10.7] [PMID: 20406067]

[140] Constantin C, Neagu M, Diana Supeanu T, Chiurciu V, A Spandidos D. IgY - turning the page toward passive immunization in COVID-19 infection (Review). Exp Ther Med 2020; 20(1): 151-8.
[http://dx.doi.org/10.3892/etm.2020.8704] [PMID: 32536989]

[141] Hamers-Casterman C, Atarhouch T, Muyldermans S, *et al.* Naturally occurring antibodies devoid of light chains. Nature 1993; 363(6428): 446-8.
[http://dx.doi.org/10.1038/363446a0] [PMID: 8502296]

[142] Arbabi-Ghahroudi M. Camelid single-domain antibodies: historical perspective and future outlook. 2017; 8(1589).

[143] Greenberg AS, Avila D, Hughes M, Hughes A, McKinney EC, Flajnik MF. A new antigen receptor gene family that undergoes rearrangement and extensive somatic diversification in sharks. Nature 1995; 374(6518): 168-73.

[http://dx.doi.org/10.1038/374168a0] [PMID: 7877689]

[144] Riechmann L, Muyldermans S. Single domain antibodies: comparison of camel VH and camelised human VH domains. J Immunol Methods 1999; 231(1-2): 25-38.
[http://dx.doi.org/10.1016/S0022-1759(99)00138-6] [PMID: 10648925]

[145] Yao H, Zhang M, Li Y, Yao J, Meng H, Yu S. Purification and quantification of heavy-chain antibodies from the milk of bactrian camels. Anim Sci J 2017; 88(9): 1446-50.
[http://dx.doi.org/10.1111/asj.12772] [PMID: 28177177]

[146] Harmsen MM, De Haard HJ. Properties, production, and applications of camelid single-domain antibody fragments. Appl Microbiol Biotechnol 2007; 77(1): 13-22.
[http://dx.doi.org/10.1007/s00253-007-1142-2] [PMID: 17704915]

[147] Könning D, Zielonka S, Grzeschik J, *et al.* Camelid and shark single domain antibodies: structural features and therapeutic potential. Curr Opin Struct Biol 2017; 45: 10-6.
[http://dx.doi.org/10.1016/j.sbi.2016.10.019] [PMID: 27865111]

[148] Chow KM, Whiteheart SW, Smiley JR, Sharma S, Boaz K, Coleman MJ, *et al.* Immunization of alpacas (Lama pacos) with protein antigens and production of antigen-specific single domain antibodies. J Vis Exp 2019; 143

[149] Leow H, Cheng Q, Fischer K, McCarthy J. The development of single domain antibodies for diagnostic and therapeutic applications. 2018.
[http://dx.doi.org/10.5772/intechopen.73324]

[150] Peyron I, Kizlik-Masson C, Dubois M-D, Atsou S, Ferrière S, Denis CV, *et al.* Camelid-derived single-chain antibodies in hemostasis: Mechanistic, diagnostic, and therapeutic applications. Research and Practice in Thrombosis and Haemostasis 2020.

[151] Vincke C, Gutiérrez C, Wernery U, Devoogdt N, Hassanzadeh-Ghassabeh G, Muyldermans S. Generation of single domain antibody fragments derived from camelids and generation of manifold constructs. Methods Mol Biol 2012; 907: 145-76.
[http://dx.doi.org/10.1007/978-1-61779-974-7_8] [PMID: 22907350]

[152] Wu Y, Jiang S, Ying T. Single-Domain Antibodies As Therapeutics against Human Viral Diseases. Front Immunol 2017; 8: 1802.
[http://dx.doi.org/10.3389/fimmu.2017.01802] [PMID: 29326699]

[153] Xiang Y, Nambulli S, Xiao Z, Liu H, Sang Z, Duprex WP, *et al.* Versatile, Multivalent Nanobody Cocktails Efficiently Neutralize SARS-CoV-2. bioRxiv : the preprint server for biology. 2020. 264333

[154] Muyldermans S. Nanobodies: natural single-domain antibodies. Annu Rev Biochem 2013; 82: 775-97.
[http://dx.doi.org/10.1146/annurev-biochem-063011-092449] [PMID: 23495938]

[155] Goldman ER, Liu JL, Zabetakis D, Anderson GP. Enhancing stability of camelid and shark single domain antibodies: An overview. Front Immunol 2017; 8: 865.
[http://dx.doi.org/10.3389/fimmu.2017.00865] [PMID: 28791022]

[156] Godakova SA, Noskov AN, Vinogradova ID, *et al.* Camelid VHHs Fused to Human Fc Fragments Provide Long Term Protection Against Botulinum Neurotoxin A in Mice. Toxins (Basel) 2019; 11(8): 464.
[http://dx.doi.org/10.3390/toxins11080464] [PMID: 31394847]

[157] Ali A, Baby B, Vijayan R. From desert to medicine: a review of camel genomics and therapeutic products. 2019; 10(17)
[http://dx.doi.org/10.3389/fgene.2019.00017]

[158] Hultberg A, Temperton NJ, Rosseels V, *et al.* Llama-derived single domain antibodies to build multivalent, superpotent and broadened neutralizing anti-viral molecules. PLoS One 2011; 6(4): e17665.
[http://dx.doi.org/10.1371/journal.pone.0017665] [PMID: 21483777]

[159] Respaud R, Vecellio L, Diot P, Heuzé-Vourc'h N. Nebulization as a delivery method for mAbs in respiratory diseases. Expert Opin Drug Deliv 2015; 12(6): 1027-39.
[http://dx.doi.org/10.1517/17425247.2015.999039] [PMID: 25557066]

[160] Larios Mora A, Detalle L, Gallup JM, *et al.* Delivery of ALX-0171 by inhalation greatly reduces respiratory syncytial virus disease in newborn lambs. MAbs 2018; 10(5): 778-95.
[http://dx.doi.org/10.1080/19420862.2018.1470727] [PMID: 29733750]

[161] Zhao G, He L, Sun S, *et al.* A Novel Nanobody Targeting Middle East Respiratory Syndrome Coronavirus (MERS-CoV) Receptor-Binding Domain Has Potent Cross-Neutralizing Activity and Protective Efficacy against MERS-CoV. J Virol 2018; 92(18): e00837-18.
[http://dx.doi.org/10.1128/JVI.00837-18] [PMID: 29950421]

[162] Stalin Raj V, Okba NMA, Gutierrez-Alvarez J, *et al.* Chimeric camel/human heavy-chain antibodies protect against MERS-CoV infection. Sci Adv 2018; 4(8): eaas9667.
[http://dx.doi.org/10.1126/sciadv.aas9667] [PMID: 30101189]

[163] Hasson S, Al-Jabri A. Immunized camels and COVID-19. 2020; 13(6): 239-41.

[164] Dong J, Huang B, Jia Z, *et al.* Development of multi-specific humanized llama antibodies blocking SARS-CoV-2/ACE2 interaction with high affinity and avidity. Emerg Microbes Infect 2020; 9(1): 1034-6.
[http://dx.doi.org/10.1080/22221751.2020.1768806] [PMID: 32403995]

[165] Dong J, Huang B, Wang B, Titong A, Kankanamalage SG, Jia Z, *et al.* Development of humanized tri-specific nanobodies with potent neutralization for SARS-CoV-2. Research Square 2020.
[http://dx.doi.org/10.1038/s41598-020-74761-y]

[166] Custódio TF, Das H, Sheward DJ, Hanke L, Pazicky S, Pieprzyk J, *et al.* Selection, biophysical and structural analysis of synthetic nanobodies that effectively neutralize SARS-CoV-2. bioRxiv 2020. 165415

[167] Li T, Cai H, Yao H, Zhou B, Zhao Y, Qin W, *et al.* Potent synthetic nanobodies against SARS-CoV-2 and molecular basis for neutralization. bioRxiv 2020. 143438

[168] Huo J, Le Bas A, Ruza RR, *et al.* Neutralizing nanobodies bind SARS-CoV-2 spike RBD and block interaction with ACE2. Nat Struct Mol Biol 2020; 27(9): 846-54.
[http://dx.doi.org/10.1038/s41594-020-0469-6] [PMID: 32661423]

[169] Gai J, Ma L, Li G, Zhu M, Qiao P, Li X, *et al.* A potent neutralizing nanobody against SARS-CoV-2 with inhaled delivery potential. bioRxiv 2020. 242867

[170] Schoof M, Faust B, Saunders RA, Sangwan S, Rezelj VV, Hoppe N, *et al.* An ultra-potent synthetic nanobody neutralizes SARS-CoV-2 by locking Spike into an inactive conformation. bioRxiv 2020. 238469

CHAPTER 4

Antiviral Potential of Immunomodulators Based Medicinal Plants against Novel Coronavirus-19: Against the Pandemic

Rinki Kumari[1,*], Bhargawi Mishra[2], Anita Venaik[3] and Snehalata Rai[4]

[1] *Department of Microbiology, Hind Institute of Medical Sciences, Mau,Ataria, Sitapur Rd, Uttar Pradesh-261303, India*

[2] *Department of Neurology, Institute of Medical Sciences, Banaras Hindu University, Uttar Pradesh-221001, India*

[3] *Department of General Management, Amity Business School, Amity University Noida Uttar Pradesh– 201313, India*

[4] *School of Biomedical Engineering, Indian Institute of Technology (Banaras Hindu University), Varanasi-221005, Uttar Pradesh, India*

Abstract: Severe acute respiratory syndrome coronavirus 2 (SARS-CoV-2) belongs to the coronavirus family and is responsible for coronavirus disease 2019 (Covid-19 is a new animal origin communicate or infectious disease). The first case of Covid19 was reported in Wuhan, China, in December 2019, and due to its rapid increase and high incidence rate, it has become a pandemic health problem worldwide. It mainly attacks the host's immune system and impairs the regulation system, playing a significant role in its pathogenesis, causing covid-19 disease. Still, we are waiting for such molecules that can act as immunomodulators and enhance the body's immune system against the disease. This literature-based chapter was prepared by searching numerous relevant SCI and SCOPUS articles on the SARS-CoV-2 and COVID-19, herbal formulation and its active molecules from different databases like- Google Scholar, PubMed, and ResearchGate. Here, we were trying to highlight or repurpose several Immunomodulators (Alkaloids, Glycosides, Flavonoids, Sapogenins, and Curcumin) of plant origin. Plant-derived Immunomodulators are capable of stimulating/suppressing the components of the host immune system and both innate and adaptive immune responses. However, in this present review, we will discuss some phytoactive chemicals, which act as immunomodulators, and their immunomodulation mechanism in the host. Hopefully, this work shall encourage the researcher community to undertake further work on plant-based antiviral therapy with potential immunomodulatory activity, which might be responsible for modulating the host immune system to cure Covid-19. Besides, we discuss the further prospect of this study.

* **Corresponding author Rinki Kumari:** Department of Microbiology, Hind Institute of Medical Sciences, Mau,Ataria, Sitapur Rd, Uttar Pradesh-261303, India; Tel: 7905101562; E-mail: rinkiv3@gmail.com

Jean-Marc Sabatier (Ed.)

Keywords: Alkaloids, COVID-19, Curcumin, Flavonoids, Glycosides, Immunomodulators, Medicinal plants, SARS-CoV-2, Sapogenins.

INTRODUCTION

In the current scenario, pandemic diseases (is known as Communicable diseases/ infectious diseases) are a major-public-health concern at the global level and are the reason for high morbidity, mortality, and transience that require extensive medical services. Due to the high rate of mutation on the viral surface, it is challenging to develop antiviral drugs or medicines that can fight against the virus or suppress its toxin effect *via* targeting viral elements. Generally, the transmission of any viral disease is spread worldwide due to travel and instant urbanization, making it a serious hazard to public health and safety [1].

Although communicable diseases (Malaria, tuberculosis, leprosy, influenza, smallpox) have played a devastating role in the past centuries, the novel coronavirus has contributed to a terrible outbreak in the 21st century, crossing several continental boundaries of the planet. However, it is closely associated with Severe Acute Respiratory Syndrome(SARS-CoV) and Middle East Respiratory Syndrome(MERS-CoV) within the human population. Symptoms including fever (high temperature), dry cough, and dyspnea are very similar to viral respiratory symptoms like flu, and its clinical features are quite similar to pneumonia [2].

Currently, it is clear that novel Covid-19 is the 3rd most dangerous animal origin pandemic disease and in 2019 first case of Covid19 was reported in Wuhan (China) with similar pneumonia symptoms (mild to moderate respiratory issues). Now, approximately 215 countries have been affected [3], and the spread has caused a high mortality rate (ranging from 100 to 100000 death so far) worldwide; however, World Health Organisation (WHO) had been declared in March 2020 that Covid19 was pandemic [4]. Continuously, cases were increasing and reached more than 23,584,259 with a high death rate (812,517), and now, SARS-CoV-2 is officially known as ICTV (International Committee on Taxonomy of Viruses), and that causes the most significant transform, globally [3, 4].

Still, covid-19 is rapidly increasing because there is no available specific treatment or drug. Therefore, we need to develop the best way to treat/manage/ prevent this infectious disease. Due to the adverse effect of chemical drugs, we still need the natural resource of Immunomodulators that can replace them in therapeutic regimens.

This study has provided better solutions in the prevention and treatment of Covid19, and some proven immunomodulators can be employed as a preventive antiviral medicine to oppose the symptoms of COVID-19. This present chapter here tries to repurpose the ancient plants' based Immunomodulators and provides a new approach for fighting the viral disease / microbial infections and their diffusion.

MATERIAL AND METHODS

Science Direct & Scopus, PubMed, Springer Link, ResearchGate, Wiley Online Library, and Google Scholar databases and Elsevier were searched, restricting the search to research articles published in English and peer-reviewed or preprint journals available. The search language rules were built with a professional librarian's guidance and included the following search terms: SARS-CoV-2, COVID-19, Medicinal plants, Immune system, Immunomodulators, Alkaloids, Glycosides, Flavonoids, Sapogenins, Curcumin and antiviral herbal formulation other- Charak Samhita, Sushrut Samhita, athar-vaveda.

The authors of this current review included recent reports, ancient literature, herbal formulation reports, and review articles. The present chapter search was conducted from May to December 2020, and obtained cited literature from various index journals was screened (from 1997 to 2020).

A GENERAL OVERVIEW ON THE NOVEL CORONA VIRUS-2019 AND ITS STRUCTURE

Genomic material of the novel coronavirus-2019 is- positive-sense single-stranded RNA virus (PSSSRNA); member of Orthocoronavirinae (includes four genera, namely alpha (α), beta (β) delta (δ) and gamma (λ) coronavirus subfamily, and the family Coronaviridae [5, 6] and mainly type α & β- CoVs infect mammals [7]. Recently, our planet found that human-affected virus family members of coronavirus -SARS-CoV-2, which have seven human-susceptible strains, mainly cause mild infections and cause severe respiratory tract infections [8].

The researcher has found a very close relationship between SARS-CoV-2 and other betaCoVs through their genomic sequencing studies. It resembles Sarbecovirus; however, 79% homology with SARS-CoV and also utilizes the same pathway as ACE2 (Angiotensin-converting enzyme 2, present on the cell of lungs, arteries, heart, *etc.*, serves as the entry point into cells for viruses) receptors to infect its hosts (human) with MERS-CoVs [8 - 10].

Some studies have defined some crucial differences between SARS-CoV-2 and other betaCoVs, making more infectious SARS-CoV; they have high transmission efficiency from human to human within a short time. SARS-CoV-2 has a primary reproduction number from other epidemic theories, denoted by R0 means transmission potential of a Cov-19-disease, *i.e.*,4.7 to 6.6 and highly infectious.

The finding has supported that these diseases' contact rate is high in the host population with the high possibility of infection, which is broadly transmitted during contact with the host [7 - 10].

The finding has defined that spherical/pleomorphic shape (Fig. **1**) of covid-19 linked with different nucleoprotein within a capsid and such a protein known as glycoprotein; makes projections on the surface that come out like a crown. Therefore, it is known as a coronavirus. Covid-19/ Cov-19 hold a different form of structural and nonstructural proteins; however, few structural proteins like a membrane (M), the envelope (E), and the spike protein (S); concerned with causing infection, cell membrane fusion, viral gathering and let lose some virus particles; induce viral genome entry into a host cell to cause infection [11]. Simultaneously, nonstructural protein induces viral replication and transcription in the host cell [12 - 14].

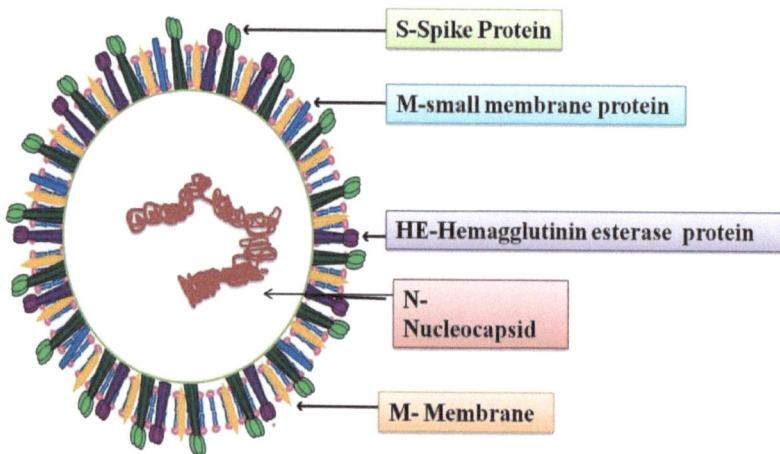

Fig. (1). The structure of Coronavirus virion with its genome RNA.

Few structural proteins (SP) have been reported to have a high affinity for causing infection, such as the spike protein (S), which is also known as a type-I transmembrane protein with a clove-shape; it comprises three parts, the first of which is a larger one known as the ectodomain (consisting of two subunits-the first subunit (S1) is a receptor-binding domain known as RBD and the second subunit (S2), the cell membrane fusion subunit); Second section, single-pass transmembrane and third, an intracellular tail.

At the initial stage of viral infection or viral pathogenesis, RBD is involved in recognizing human host cell receptors; after recognition, the interaction between the host cell and S proteins of the virus forms a bond among RBD and host cell receptors and that cause cross-species transmission. Several studies have been found that HCov-19 (HumanCoV) recognized different types of host cell receptors like human aminopeptidase N (hAPN) (host cell receptors) identified by HCoV-229E [15] other dipeptidyl peptidase-4 (DPP4) identified by MERS-CoV (Dipeptidyl peptidase 4 is a functional receptor for the emerging human coronavirus-EMC [16].

Other most crucial host cell receptors are angiotensin-converting enzyme 2 (ACE2) or human angiotensin-converting enzyme 2 (hACE2) that recognized only by SARS-CoV S protein and only after utilization of Transmembrane Serine Protease 2 (TMPRSS2), coronavirus can enter the host cell then use host replication machinery for causing infection or disease. Therefore, the studies have proved that spike-S glycoprotein possess a greater binding affinity with ACE2 and might also be responsible for greater pathogenicity of -CoV-2 as it also occurs in the highly infectious form of the virus [17]

The researcher also identified that humans' respiratory tracts comprise several ACE2 receptors and increase vulnerability to coronavirus and is one of the reasons for the rapidly increasing incidence rate of Covid-19 globally. After the virus's genome enters the host cell, it can initiate the subsequent inflammatory mechanism and induced/promote to release of various pro-inflammatory cytokines (like G-CSF, IP-10, MCP-1, MIP-1a, IL-2, IL-7, IL-10, and TNF-α) cause inflammation. Recently, some case studies have reported a high level of pro-inflammatory cytokines found in the severe case of Covid-19 patients [16 - 18].

IMMUNSYSTEM AND IMMONOMODULATORS

It is well known that the body has its natural fighting system against different microbial or communicated agents or diseases, called immunity, and some are a factor such infectious agents, immunization-vaccine, and several external stimuli (act as an inducer) are also able to initiate or induced/ trigger immune-system of body. This is a significant facet of immunity capable of distinguishing between the body's proteins or molecules or cells and foreign entities/molecules. Another way, the body's immune system recognizes foreign particles when entering the host cell; then collective and coordinate rejoinder with specific cells, mediate mechanism against the foreign particles and trigger the foreign cell [18].

As shown in Fig. (2) the body's immune system's function has been categorized into the section-1) Innate immune system/nonspecific immune system-the microbio-logical, chemical, and physical barriers; 2) Adaptive immune system/ specific or acquired immune system.

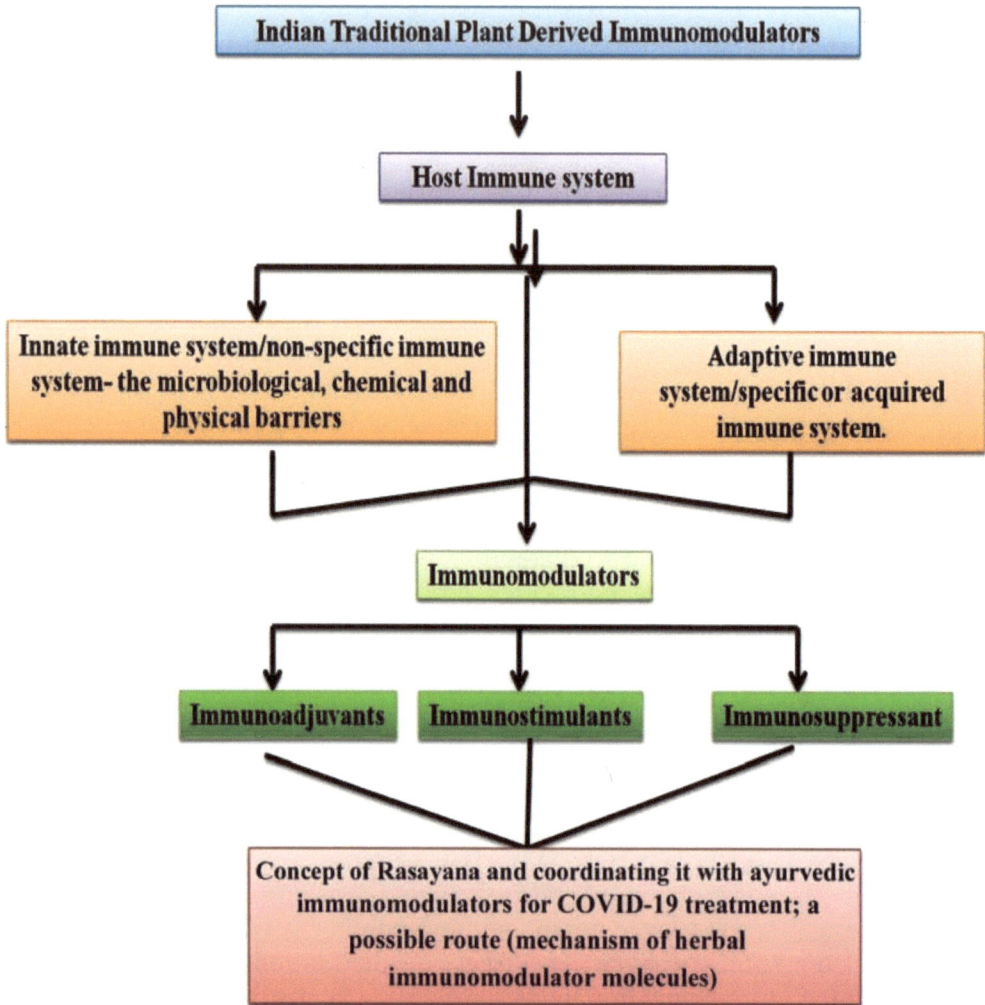

Fig. (2). Systematic presentation of host immune system with the possible route of herbal Immunomo-dulators.

Host immune system can recognize several pathogens by the presence of pathogen-associated molecular patterns (PAMPs) through sensor- pattern recognition receptors (PRRs)(belong to DNA receptors – (cytosolic sensors for DNA), NOD-like receptors, RIG-I-like receptors, and toll-like receptors) [19, 20]; and instantly fighting system of body release or induce secretion of the various pro-inflammatory maker - cytokines, acute phase proteins, chemokines, type I interferons, macrophages, monocytes, complement, and neutrophils; able to trigger pathogen at the time [19]. However, the immune system (IS) is always sustained homeostasis within the host body and the efficiency of IS, affected by some factors, are exogenous and endogenous, and responsible for immuno-suppression/ immunostimulation; Such molecules normalize/modulate the pathophysiological mechanism known as immunomodulators [20 - 24].

These immunomodulators may be natural or synthetic molecules classified as immunoadjuvants (act as immune stimulators and improve vaccine efficacy), immunostimulants (act as immune system activators/ inducers), immuno-suppressants; capable of modulating, suppressing, and stimulating all forms of IS. Though immunosuppressants inhibit the IS and control the pathological immune response consequent to organ transplantation, these agents are useful in treating a communicated disease or autoimmune diseases. There are various monoclonal antibodies, and chemically synthesized molecules prepared, which act as immunomodulators. Consequently, immunomodulatory agents are essential to trigger pathogens; still, they will be required with additional safety and efficiency [25].

According to reports, host's IS plays a significant role in the treatment and spreading of covid-19 infection. So that from the previous finding, herbal immunomodulators have a potential effect in the prevention and treatment of Covid-19 because herbal immunomodulators contain several bioactive molecules-phytochemicals, possess antimicrobial, antiviral, anti-inflammatory, and immunostimulatory activities (to modulate the immune response) such as, plant-derived immunomodulators compounds – alkaloids, glycosides, flavonoids, sapogenins, and curcumin, *etc.*

CONCEPT OF RASAYANA AND RELATIONSHIP BETWEEN HERBAL IMMUNOMODULATORS WITH AYURVEDA FOR COVID19 TREATMENT, A POSSIBLE ROUTE

Various reports provide the popularity and demand of the Ayurvedic medicine system (which is the oldest traditional medical organization) because it is more effective and protects various microbial effects or communicated diseases since the Vedic period 1500-500BCE (Fig. **3**) [21 - 24]. Natural-based medicine's significant role has been explained in the *athar-vaveda* (before 1200BC), *Charak Samhita*, and *Sushrut Samhita* (1000e500BC) and are the essential classic proven literature where one could find all details about medicinal herbs. This ancient health care system has specific and well-defined management and treatment for each and every type of disease. In the Indian therapeutic system, two central medical practices had arisen for curing the wide range of microbial/infectious diseases [27, 28].

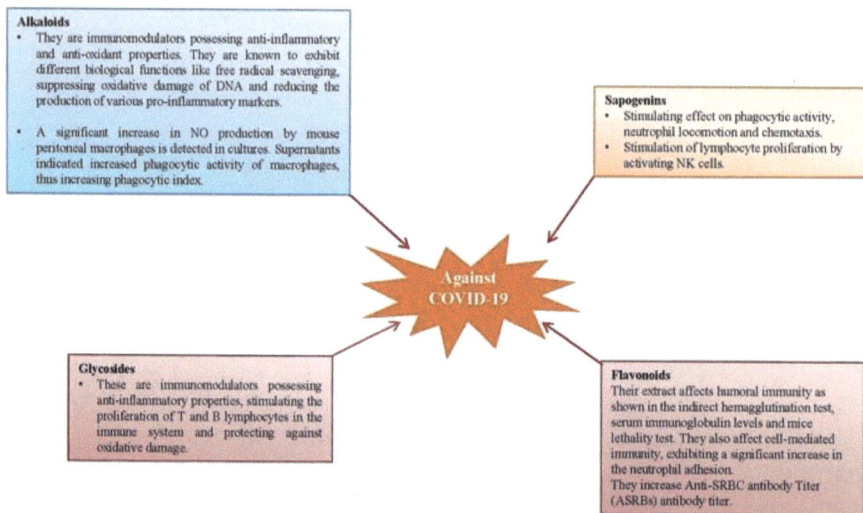

Alkaloids
- They are immunomodulators possessing anti-inflammatory and anti-oxidant properties. They are known to exhibit different biological functions like free radical scavenging, suppressing oxidative damage of DNA and reducing the production of various pro-inflammatory markers.
- A significant increase in NO production by mouse peritoneal macrophages is detected in cultures. Supernatants indicated increased phagocytic activity of macrophages, thus increasing phagocytic index.

Sapogenins
- Stimulating effect on phagocytic activity, neutrophil locomotion and chemotaxis.
- Stimulation of lymphocyte proliferation by activating NK cells.

Against COVID-19

Glycosides
- These are immunomodulators possessing anti-inflammatory properties, stimulating the proliferation of T and B lymphocytes in the immune system and protecting against oxidative damage.

Flavonoids
Their extract affects humoral immunity as shown in the indirect hemagglutination test, serum immunoglobulin levels and mice lethality test. They also affect cell-mediated immunity, exhibiting a significant increase in the neutrophil adhesion.
They increase Anti-SRBC antibody Titer (ASRBs) antibody titer.

Fig. (3). Repurpose some herbal Immunomodulators acting against Covid-19.

Rasayana is the Ayurvedic word and formed by combining two comments, Rasa + Andayana, meaning nutrition and carrying in the body, and ayurveda medicine system is recognized as *Rasayana therapy* (RT). RT is capable of enhancing the qualities of life with longevity, better memory power, and intelligence, liberty from mental or other disorders. As a dedicated torrent of traditional medication for immune promotion, anti-neuro-degenerative and rejuvenating health care can prevent the effects of aging. RT is playing a significant role in the improvement of immunity [29].

Various studies observed that there are various plants based immunomodulators or immune-molecules (Table **1**) [30 - 53], used in the Rasayana therapy that attracts attention of community and researcher, world-wide; because of several natural immunomodulators, perform immunomodulatory action on deadly infectious diseases.

Table 1. A list of common plant-derived Immunomodulators with their pharmacology activity.

Plant/Family Name	Ayurvedics/Common Name	Plant Part Used	Phytoactive Molecules	Mechanism of Biological Activities
Ocimum sanctum Linn. (Labiateae)	Tulshi	Entire part	Oils - eugenol, cavacrol, derivatives of ursolic acid, apigenin	Stimulatory effect on humoral immunity that involved in immune system [30]

(Table 1) cont.....

Plant/Family Name	Ayurvedics/Common Name	Plant Part Used	Phytoactive Molecules	Mechanism of Biological Activities
Morus alba Linn. (Moraceae)	Brahmdaru	Fruits, leaves, bark	Flavonoids, anthocyanins	Regulate humoral immunity and also cell-mediated immunity, showing significant increase in the neutrophil adhesion [31]
Aloe vera Tourn.ex Linn. (Liliaceae)	Kumaari	Gel from leaves	Anthraquinone glycosides	Act as immunostimulation due to activation of macrophages [32 - 34]
Andrographis paniculata Nees (Acanthaceae)	Kaalmegha	Leaves	Leaves Diterpenes	Acts as inhibitor of TNF-α Induces significant stimulation of both "antigen specific" and Antigen nonspecific [35]
Asparagus racemosus Wild. (Liliaceae)	Shatavaari	Roots	Saponins, sitosterols	Act as immunoadjuvant Regulate immune system and protective cell [36]
Murraya koenigii (L) Spreng. (Rutaceae)	Surabhini-nimba	Leaves	Coumarin, carbazole alkaloids, glucoside	Act as immunostimulation *in vitro* and *in vivo*. Elevate the production of NO Increase phagocytic activity of macrophages thus increase in phagocytic index by rapid removal of carbon particles from blood stream [37]
Couroupita guianensis Aubl. (Lecythidaceae)	Nagalinga	Fruits, flowers	Steroids, flavonoids, phenolics	Followed immunostimulation *in vitro* and *in vivo* Increased phagocytic activity [38]
Tinospora cordifolia Miers. (Menispermiaceae)	Amrita, guduuchii	Entire herb	Alkaloidal constituents such as berberine, tinosporic acid	Improves the phagocyte function without affecting both immune systems Acts as immunomodulatorp [39]
Lagenaria siceraria Mol. (Cucurbitaceae)	Katu-tumbi	Leaves, fruit	Cucurbitacin, beta-glycosidase	Extract showed immunostimulation *in vitro* and *in vivo* by increasing the DTH [40]

(Table 1) cont.....

Plant/Family Name	Ayurvedics/Common Name	Plant Part Used	Phytoactive Molecules	Mechanism of Biological Activities
Terminalia arjuna Roxb. (Combretaceae)	Arjuna	Leaves, bark	Flavonoids, oligomeric proanthocyanidins, tannins	Plant showed immunomodulation by increasing the secondary immune response as evidenced by an increase in Anti- SRBC antibody titre (ASRBs) antibody titer but failed to modulate primary immune response [41]
Bauhinia variegata Linn. (Caesalpiniaceae)	Kaanchana	Roots, bark, buds	Flavonoids, beta-sitosterol, lupeol	Increase in macrophage stimulatory activity, Act as immunomodulatory potential [42]
Urena lobata Linn. (Malvaceae)	Naagabala	Roots, flowers	Flavanoids	Immunostimulation action Increased phagocytic activity [43]
Gymnema sylvestre R.Br. (Asclepiadaceae)	Gurmaar	Leaves	Sapogenins	Extract showed significant immunomodulation at all concentrations in various *in vitro* models by exerting a stimulating effect on phagocytic activity, neutrophil locomotion and chemotaxis [44]
Cordia superba Cham. and *C. rufescens* A. DC. (Boraginaceae)	Shleshmaataka	Leaf, fruit, bark	Alpha-amyrin	Extract showed a significant immunomodulation by stimulating the NO, IFN-γ and lipopolysaccharide [45]
Cissampelos pareira Linn. (Menispermiaceae)	Paatha	Roots	Hayatine alkaloids	Stimulates immune system, affects humoral immunity as shown by its effect in the indirect hemagglutination test, serum immunoglobulin levels. It also affects cell-mediated immunity [46]
Alternanthera tenella Colla (Amaranthaceae)	Snow Ball	Herb	Flavonoids, triterpenes	Immunostimulation through modulation of B-lymphocyte functions was achieved using aqueous extracts of *A. tenella* [47]

(Table 1) cont.....

Plant/Family Name	Ayurvedics/Common Name	Plant Part Used	Phytoactive Molecules	Mechanism of Biological Activities
Ganoderma lucidum (Fr.) P. Karst. (Polyporaceae)	Reishi mushroom	Whole plant	Flavonoids, triterpenes	Induction of cytokine (TNF-α, IFN-γ) by *Ganoderma* suggests its immunomodulatory potential [48]
Nyctanthes arbor-tristis L. (Oleaceae)	Paarijaata	Leaf, seeds	Iridoid glucosides	Potentially stimulates immune system and affects both humoral immunity as well as cell-mediated immunity as shown by its effect in the indirect hemagglutination test and serum immunoglobulin levels [49]
Actinidia macrosperma (Actinidiaceae)	Actinidia	Fruits	Alkaloids, saponins	Acts as Immunomodulator by lymphocyte proliferation stimulation and by activating NK cells [50]
Boswellia spp. (Burseraceae)	Shallaki	Gum resin	Triterpenes, ursanes	Stimulatory effect on lymphocyte proliferation [51]
Hyptis suaveolens (L.) Poit., (Lamaceae)	Tumbaaka	Leaf, flowers	Lupeol, beta-sitosterol	Potentially suppresses immune system affecting both humoral immunity and cell-mediated immunity as shown by its effect in indirect hemagglutination test [52]
Allium hirtifolium Boiss. (Alliaceae)	Persian shallot	Herb	Thiosulfinates, flavonoids	Increase in footpad thickness due to immunomodulatory activity [53]
Citrus natsudaidai Hayata (Rutaceae)	Japanese summer grape fruit	Fruits	Auraptene, flavonoids	Immunostimulatory effect on lymphocyte proliferation, induction of cytokine (TNF-α, INF-γ) [48]

ALKALOIDS

Alkaloid is an organic compound that isolates from a natural source and is also prepared through synthetic derivation. Based on its chemistry, it is necessary and comprises 1 or 2 nitrogen atoms. Generally, it is heterocyclic and found in different plants like *Achillea millefolium, Murraya koenigii, Cissampelos pareira,* and *Actinidia macrosperma.* Several studies have shown that alkaloid (secondary metabolites) act as immunomodulator and possess anti-inflammatory, antioxidant agents. It is known to exhibit different biological functions like free radical scavenging, suppress oxidative damage of DNA, and reduced the production of various pro-inflammatory markers [54, 55].

GLYCOSIDES

It is a phytochemical compound and acts as plant-derived immunomodulatory and the acetals/ sugar ethers, made by the interaction of the hydroxyl groups (OH)of the sugar non-sugar moieties, with the loss of a water molecule (H_2O). They are present in different plants with different forms (iridoid glycosides) like *Aloe Vera Tourn. ex Linn. (Liliaceae), Mollugo verticillata L. (Molluginaceae),* and *Picrorhiza scrophulariiflora Benth. (Scrophulariaceae),* that possess antioxidant, immunomodulator, and anti-inflammatory. This can stimulate the proliferation of T and B lymphocytes in the immune system and protect them from oxidative damage [49, 56].

FLAVONOIDS

Flavonoids (polyphenolic -plant secondary metabolites) are found in *Terminalia arjuna, Morus alba Linn. (Moraceae), Murraya koenigii (L) Spreng. (Rutaceae), Achillea millefolium C. Koch (Compositae)* and *Alternanthera tenella Colla (Amaranthaceae) etc.* It has a different pharmacological activity like antifungal, astringent, antitumor, anti-inflammatory, and antiviral and also exert immunomodulatory activities because of the diverse form of flavonoids like flavones, flavonols, isoflavones, flavonols, flavanones, flavanonols, and chalcones [57, 58]. Its chemical structure has a 15 carbon skeleton -C6- C3-C6- and consists of 2 phenyl rings connected by a 3-carbon bridge [59]. Some studies suggested that flavonoids can suppress pro-inflammatory activity and induce the T regulatory subset of the immune system. During the mechanism, some different flavonoids can reduce the production of immunoglobulin E and modulate the expression of Th2 cytokines with other cytokines like IL-4 and IL-5. Flavonoids reduced these cytokines level (otherwise switching immunoglobulin E). Activated mast cells produced different chemical mediators (PGD2, mMCPT-1 Cys-L, and TSLP), leading to the targeting of pathogens. However, some other finding supported that they have an inhibitory effect on the cytotoxic lymphocyte activity and also inhibit the production of IL-6 production, thereby, having a potential role as immunomodulators (immune system responses), balancing Th1/Th2 in the immune system [60 - 65].

SAPOGENINS

Sapogenins are also secondary metabolites found in the *Gymnema Sylvestre, Chlorophytum borivilianum, Boswellia spp.,* and *Randia dumetorum*. Different forms of sapogenins like triterpenoid saponins and diterpenes possess a wide range of biological or pharmacological activity, including immunomodulatory activities [66].

CURCUMIN

Curcumin is an organic compound found in the *Curcuma longa* (C. longa) or turmeric, known as rhizomatous; it belongs to *Zingiberaceae* and genus Curcuma [67]. Generally, turmeric is the king of kitchen as a spice, a natural yellow color, and flavor. From the ancient period, turmeric is an essential herbal medicine in the Indian Ayurveda medicinal system. It has been used to treat various diseases (management of obesity, diabetes mellitus, asthma, cardiovascular and inflammatory bowel disease) [S. Hewlings]. This contains major important photo-active compounds like curcuminoid (curcumin), demethoxycurcumin, and bisdemethoxycurcumin, besides carbohydrates, protein, fat, and minerals. Due to the presence of these active compounds, it possesses antioxidant, anti-neurodegenerative, anti-inflammatory, and anti-cancer properties [68].

The study demonstrated that curcumin significantly controls blood pressure by decreasing angiotensin II receptor type 1 (AT1). Curcumin can control hypertension (is one symptom of covid19 patients), and in this case, the expression of angiotensin-converting enzyme (ACE) increases. Therefore, it is proved that curcumin acts as an antihypertension agent and follows a mechanism like that of ACE inhibitor agents, which inhibits the expression or activity of ACE and activates a feedback process and can increase the amount of ACE to maintain body homeostasis [69 - 73].

Another finding also supports its anti-inflammatory action, and this action is governed by inhibition on the toll-like receptors 4 (TLR-4), phosphatidylinositol-3 kinase (PI3K), nuclear factor-kappa B (NF-κB) or also regulate the expression of these receptors. Another hand decreases the formation of different pro-inflammatory cytokines like IL-6, interleukin Beta (IL-1β), and tumor necrosis factor-alpha (TNFα) [71 - 74], whereas some other evidence has supported both nature immunostimulation and immune-suppression [74]. Therefore, on this basis, this evidence can repurpose the curcumin for the treatment of Covid19 patients. A more detailed investigation is urgently needed to elucidate the effect of curcumin effect in the treatment and prevention of this communicated disease. Further, extensive research is required to validate herbal immunomodulators and their molecular mechanisms in *in-silico*, pre-clinical, and well-designed clinical trials.

It would be interesting to design future therapeutic approaches for immunomo-dulatory pathways with a synergistic combination of natural herbal drugs.

CONCLUSION

In short, COVID-19 is a kind of animal-origin respiratory disease, affecting mainly the weak immune system for spreading the pathogenesis of this disease. It was also declared that it affects only the respiratory part of the body, affecting the host's body, and for this responsible virus is severe acute respiratory syndrome coronavirus 2 [SARS-CoV-2] that also impaired the quality of life. SARS-CoV-2 highly impairs the immune system of host cells; only those who have a robust immune system can survive. There is no clinical element or medicine, either vaccine or drug, available to treat this covid19; only some supportive management like hand sanitization repeat after 20 seconds, make the distance, and wearing full mouth mask, possibly can prevent the transmission of the virus.

Globally, several researchers and communities are being tried to perform to discover such an alternative source to find out for better cure way. Some selected herbal molecules are in the clinical trial phase but still have not reached the goal; they take more time for final approval. This type of pandemics is already explained in the Indian tradition ancient era called epidemics or Janapadodhwamsaand, from ancient period various herbal-based medicine have well suppressed or prevented the pandemic disease.

This herbal medicine can re-regulate the immune system of the host cell and improve the immunomodulatory process. These herbal-derived immunomo-dulators are capable of reducing the production of different pro-inflammatory markers. Work has proven its benefits to be utilized for the prevention and cure of these pandemics. Naturally, several existing herbal medicines could act as immunomodulators for the treatment of Covid19.

This summarizes information concerning the phyto-active biomolecules, biological, chemistry, and cellular activities and the clinical prospect of plants derived immunomodulators to provide sufficient baseline scientific information that could help discover plant-based medicine providing new functional leads for coronavirus. Therefore, here, the critically reviewed concept of Rasāyana defines how immunomodulators modulate the immune system or promote free radical scavenger mechanisms to protect cells and boost up the immune system.

In short, we all are aware that COVID-19 has entered a dangerous or unsafe phase, creating destruction in human society and every society of the universe, thus leading to enhanced globalization. Still, there are no safe drugs, vaccines, and therapeutics available against unabated transmission of covid 19.

Our research focuses on formulating such drugs/medicines from the natural alternative sources that prevent adverse effects. In the future, we need extensive research to formulate herbal-based immunomodulators and detect their molecular mechanisms and extension to a broad spectrum of a different phase of a clinical trial. It is also exciting to plan future therapeutic approaches for an immunomodulatory mechanism with a synergistic combination of natural herbal drugs. However, the molecular pathway and interaction of herbal immunomodulators with different pro-inflammatory markers can be used in future immunotherapeutic strategies.

CONSENT FOR PUBLICATION

Not applicable.

CONFLICT OF INTEREST

The authors declare no conflict of interest, financial or otherwise.

ACKNOWLEDGEMENTS

Declared none.

AUTHORS CONTRIBUTION

The present chapter was carried out with the collaboration with all the authors, and they have fully contributed to this chapter planed, preparation, and editing of the same.

REFERENCES

[1]   Ahmad A, Rehman MU, Alkharfy KM. An alternative approach to minimize the risk of coronavirus (Covid-19) and similar infections. Eur Rev Med Pharmacol Sci 2020; 24(7): 4030-4. [PMID: 32329879]

[2]   Morawska L, Cao J. Airborne transmission of SARS-CoV-2: The world should face the reality. Environ Int 2020; 139: 105730. [http://dx.doi.org/10.1016/j.envint.2020.105730] [PMID: 32294574]

[3]   Acharya KP. Resource poor countries ought to focus on early detection and containment of novel corona virus at the point of entry. Clin Epidemiol Glob Health 2020. [http://dx.doi.org/10.1016/j.cegh.2020.03.001] [PMID: 32292836]

[4]   Gautret P, Lagier JC, Parola P, *et al.* Hydroxychloroquine and azithromycin as a treatment of COVID-19: results of an open-label non-randomized clinical trial. Int J Antimicrob Agents 2020; 56(1): 105949. [http://dx.doi.org/10.1016/j.ijantimicag.2020.105949] [PMID: 32205204]

[5]   Huang C, Wang Y, Li X, *et al.* Clinical features of patients infected with 2019 novel coronavirus in Wuhan, China. Lancet 2020; 395(10223): 497-506.
[http://dx.doi.org/10.1016/S0140-6736(20)30183-5] [PMID: 31986264]

[6]   Gorbalenya AE, *et al.* Coronaviridae Study Group of the International Committee on Taxonomy of Viruses. The species Severe acute respiratory syndrome-related coronavirus: classifying 2019-nCoV and naming it SARS-CoV-2. Nat Microbiol 2020; 5(4): 536-44.
[http://dx.doi.org/10.1038/s41564-020-0695-z] [PMID: 32123347]

[7]   Fan Y, Zhao K, Shi ZL, Zhou P. Bat Coronaviruses in China. Viruses 2019; 11(3): 210.
[http://dx.doi.org/10.3390/v11030210] [PMID: 30832341]

[8]   Hewlings SJ, Kalman DS. Curcumin: a review of its' effects on human health. Foods 2017; 6(10): 1-11.
[http://dx.doi.org/10.3390/foods6100092] [PMID: 29065496]

[9]   Guo YR, Cao QD, Hong ZS, *et al.* The origin, transmission and clinical therapies on coronavirus disease 2019 (COVID-19) outbreak - an update on the status. Mil Med Res 2020; 7(1): 11.
[http://dx.doi.org/10.1186/s40779-020-00240-0] [PMID: 32169119]

[10]   Peng X, Xu X, Li Y, Cheng L, Zhou X, Ren B. Transmission routes of 2019- nCoV and controls in dental practice. Int J Oral Sci 2020; 12(1): 9.
[http://dx.doi.org/10. 1038/s41368-020-0075-9]

[11]   Zhang YZ, Holmes EC. A genomic perspective on the origin and emergence of SARS-CoV-2. Cell 2020; 181(2): 223-7.
[http://dx.doi.org/10.1016/j.cell.2020.03.035] [PMID: 32220310]

[12]   Zhang T, Wu Q, Zhang Z. Probable pangolin origin of SARS-CoV-2 associated with the COVID-19 outbreak. Curr Biol 2020; 30(7): 1346-51.
[http://dx.doi.org/10.1016/j.cub.2020.03.022.e2]

[13]   Hamming I, Timens W, Bulthuis ML, Lely AT, Navis G, van Goor H. Tissue distribution of ACE2 protein, the functional receptor for SARS coronavirus. A first step in understanding SARS pathogenesis. J Pathol 2004; 203(2): 631-7.
[http://dx.doi.org/10.1002/path.1570] [PMID: 15141377]

[14]   Li F . Structure, function, and evolution of coronavirus spike proteins. Annu Rev Virol 2016; 29; 3(1): 237-61.

[15]   Lan J, Ge J, Yu J, *et al.* Structure of the SARS-CoV-2 spike receptor-binding domain bound to the ACE2 receptor. Nature 2020; 581(7807): 215-20.
[http://dx.doi.org/10.1038/s41586-020-2180-5] [PMID: 32225176]

[16]   Wrapp D, Wang N, Corbett KS, *et al.* Cryo-EM structure of the 2019-nCoV spike in the prefusion conformation. Science 2020; 13; 367(6483): 1260-3.

[17]   Snijder EJ, Decroly E, Ziebuhr J. The Nonstructural Proteins Directing Coronavirus RNA Synthesis and Processing. Adv Virus Res 2016; 96: 59-126.
[http://dx.doi.org/10.1016/bs.aivir.2016.08.008] [PMID: 27712628]

[18]   Wentworth DE, Holmes KV. Molecular determinants of species specificity in the coronavirus receptor aminopeptidase N (CD13): influence of N-linked glycosylation. J Virol 2001; 75(20): 9741-52.
[http://dx.doi.org/10.1128/JVI.75.20.9741-9752.2001] [PMID: 11559807]

[19]   Raj VS, Mou H, Smits SL, *et al.* Dipeptidyl peptidase 4 is a functional receptor for the emerging human coronavirus-EMC. Nature 2013; 14; 495(7440): 251-4.
[http://dx.doi.org/10.1038/nature12005]

[20]   Hofmann H, Pyrc K, van der Hoek L, Geier M, Berkhout B, Pöhlmann S. Human coronavirus NL63 employs the severe acute respiratory syndrome coronavirus receptor for cellular entry. Proc Natl Acad Sci USA 2005; 31; 102(22): 7988-93.

[http://dx.doi.org/10.1073/pnas.0409465102]

[21]   Baxter D. Active and passive immunity, vaccine types, excipients and licensing. Occup Med (Lond) 2007; 57(8): 552-6.
       [http://dx.doi.org/10.1093/occmed/kqm110] [PMID: 18045976]

[22]   Ford MS, Roach SS. Introductory clinical pharmacology. 27th ed.. USA: Lippincott Williams and Wilkins 2009; p. 567e568.

[23]   Hofmeyr SA. An interpretative introduction to the immune system. In: Cohen I, Segel L, Eds. Design Principles for the Immune System and other Distributed Autonomous Systems. NY, USA: Oxford University Press, Inc 2001; p. 3e24.

[24]   Parkin J, Cohen B. An overview of the immune system. Lancet 2001; 357(9270): 1777-89.
       [http://dx.doi.org/10.1016/S0140-6736(00)04904-7] [PMID: 11403834]

[25]   El-Sheikh ALK. Renal Transport and Drug Interactions of Immunosuppressants. Nijmegen, Netherlands: Radbound University 2008; p. 62.

[26]   Chulet R, Pradhan P. A review on rasayana. Phcog Rev 2010; 3(6): 229e34.

[27]   Dahanukar SA, Thatte UM. Current status of ayurveda in phytomedicine. Phytomedicine 1997; 4(4): 359-68.
       [http://dx.doi.org/10.1016/S0944-7113(97)80048-7] [PMID: 23195589]

[28]   Bhattacharya SK, Bhattacharya A, Chakrabarti A. Adaptogenic activity of Siotone, a polyherbal formulation of Ayurvedic rasayanas. Indian J Experimental Biol 2000; 38: 119e28.

[29]   Vaghasiya J, Datani M, Nandkumar K, Malaviya S, Jivani N. Comparative evaluation of alcoholic and aqueous extracts of Ocimum sanctum for immunomodulatory activity. Int J Pharm Biol Res 2010; 1(1): 25e9.

[30]   Bharani SER, Asad M, Dhamanigi SS, Chandrakala GK. Immunomodulatory activity of methanolic extract of Morus alba linn. (mulberry) leaves. Pak J Pharm Sci 2010; 23(1): 63e8.

[31]   Sikarwar Mukesh S, Patil MB, Shalini S. Aloe vera: plant of immortality. IJPSR 2010; 1: 7e10.

[32]   Hamman JH. Composition and applications of Aloe vera leaf gel. Molecules 2008; 13: 1599e616.
       [http://dx.doi.org/10.3390/molecules13081599]

[33]   Cooper JC, Turcasso N. Immunostimulatory effects of b-1,3 glucan and acemannan. 1999; JANA 2: 5e11.

[34]   Varma A, Padh H, Shrivastava N. Andrographolide: a new plant-derived antineoplastic entity on horizon. Evid Based Complement Alternat Med 2011; 2011: 815390.
       [http://dx.doi.org/10.1093/ecam/nep135] [PMID: 19752167]

[35]   Bopana N, Saxena S. Asparagus racemosusdethnopharmacological evaluation and conservation needs. J Ethnopharmacol 2007; 110: 1e15.

[36]   Shah SA, Wakade AS, Juvekr AR. Immunomodulatory activity methanolic extract of Murraya koenigii (L) Spreng. leaves. Indian J Exp Biol 2007; 46: 505e9.

[37]   Pradhan D, Panda PK, Tripathy G. Evaluation of immunomodulatory activity of methanolic extract of Couroupita guianensis Aubl flowers in rat. NPR 2009; 8(1): 37e42.

[38]   Sinha K, Mishra NP, Singh J, Kanjua SPS. Tinospora cordifolia, a reservoir plant for therapeutic applications: A review. IJTK 2004; 3(3): 257e70.

[39]   Deshpande JR, Choudhary AA, Mirsha MR, Meghre VS, Wadokar SG, Dorle AK. Benefical effects of *Lagenaria siceraria* Mol.. Fruit epicarp in animal models. Indian J Exp Biol 2008; 46: 234e42..

[40]   Halder S, Bharal N, Mediratta PK, Kaur I, Sharma KK. Anti-inflammatory, Immunomodulatory and anti-nociceptic activity of Terminalia arjuna Roxb. Bark powder in mice and rats. Indian J Exp Biol 2009; 47: 577e83.

[41] Ghaisas MM, Saikh SA, Deshpande AD. Evaluation of immunomodulatory activity of ethanolic extract of stem bark of Bauhinia variegata Linn. IJGP 2009; 3(1): 70e4.

[42] Rinku M, Prasanth VV, Parthasarathy G. Immunomodulatory activity of the methanolic extract of Urena lobata Linn. Int J Pharmacol 2009; 7: 1.http://www.ispub.com/journal/the_internet_journal_of_pharmacology/volume_7_number_1_27/article/ immunomodulatory-activity-of-the-methanolic-extract-ofurena-lobata-linn.html

[43] Malik JK, Manvi FV, Nanjwade BK, Alagawadi KR, Sinsh S. Immunomodulatory activity of Gymnema sylvestre R.Br. leaves on *in vitro* human neutrophils. J Pharm Res 2009; 2(8): 1284e6.

[44] Costa JFO, David JPL, David JM, *et al.* Immunomodulatory activity of extracts from Cordia superba Cham. and Cordia rufescens A. DC. (Boraginaceae), plant species native from Brazilian semiarid. Rev Bras Farmaacogn 2008; 18(1): 11e5.

[45] Bafna A, Mishra S. Antioxidant and immunomodulatory activity of the alkaloidal fraction of Cissampelos pareira Linn. O‟PhG 2009; 78: 21e31.

[46] Guerra RNM, Pereira HAW, Silveria LMS, Olea RSG. Evaluation of immunomodulatory and anti-inflammatory effects and phytochemical screening of Alternanthera tenella Colla (Amaranthaceae) aqueous extract. Braz J Med Biol Res 2003; 36: 1215e9.

[47] Habijanic J, Berovic M, Wraber B, Hodzar D, Boh B. Immunostimulatory effects of fungal polysaccharides from Ganoderma lucidum submerged biomass cultivation. Food Technol Biotechnol 2001; 39(9): 327e31.

[48] Kannan M, Ranjit Singh AJA, Ajith Kumar TT, Jegatheswari P, Subburayalu S. Studies on immuno-bioactivities of Nyctanthes arbortristis (Oleaceae). Afr J Microbiol Res 2007; 1(6): 88e91.

[49] Lu Y, Fan J, Zhao Y, *et al.* Immunomodulatory activity of aqueous extract of Actinidia macrosperma. Asia Pac J Clin Nutr 2007; 16(1): 261e5.

[50] Mikhaeil BR, Maatooq G, Badria T, Farid AA, Mohamed MA. Chemistry and immunomodulatory activity of frankincense oil. J Chem Sci 2002; 58: 230e8.

[51] Jain V, Bhagwat D, Jat RC, Bhardwaj S. The immunomodulation potential of Hyptis suaveolens. IJPRD 2005; 1(11): 1e6.

[52] Tanaka T, Sugiura H, Inaba R, *et al.* Immunomodulatory action of Citrus auraptene on macrophage functions and cytokine production of lumphocytes in female BALB/c mice. Carcinogenesis 1999; 20(8): 1471e6.

[53] Kokate CK, Purohit AP, Gokhale SB. Pharmacognosy. Mumbai: Nirali Prakashan 2004.

[54] Calis I, Yuruker A, Tasdemir D, Wright AD, Sticher O, Pezzuto JM. Cycloartan triterpine glycosides from the root of Astragalus melanophrurius. Planta Med 1997; 63: 183e6.

[55] Cherng JM, Chiang W, Chiang LC. Immunomodulatory activities of common vegetables and spices of Umbelliferae and its related coumarins and flavonoids. Food Chem 2007; 106(3): 944e50.

[56] Chang SL, Chiang YM, Chang CLT, *et al.* Flavonoids, centaurein and centaureidin, from Bidens pilosa, stimulate IFN expression. J Ethnopharmacol 2007; 112: 232e6.

[57] Ito T, Warnken SP, May WS. Protein synthesis inhibition by flavonoids: roles of eukaryotic initiation factor 2alpha kinases. Biochem Biophys Res Commun 1999; 265(2): 589-94. [http://dx.doi.org/10.1006/bbrc.1999.1727] [PMID: 10558914]

[58] Kang SR, Park KI, Park HS, Lee DH, Kim JA, Nagappan A. Anti-inflammatory effect of flavonoids isolated from Korea Citrus aurantium L. on lipopolysaccharide-induced mouse macrophage RAW 264.7 cells by blocking of nuclear factor-kappa B (NF-κB) and mitogen-activated protein kinase (MAPK) signalling pathways. Food Chem 2011; 129: 1721-8. [http://dx.doi.org/10.1016/j.foodchem.2011.06.039]

[59] Hougee S, Sanders A, Faber J, *et al.* Decreased pro-inflammatory cytokine production by LPS-stimulated PBMC upon *in vitro* incubation with the flavonoids apigenin, luteolin or chrysin, due to selective elimination of monocytes/macrophages. Biochem Pharmacol 2005; 69(2): 241-8.
[http://dx.doi.org/10.1016/j.bcp.2004.10.002] [PMID: 15627476]

[60] Middleton E Jr, Kandaswami C, Theoharides TC. The effects of plant flavonoids on mammalian cells: implications for inflammation, heart disease, and cancer. Pharmacol Rev 2000; 52(4): 673-751.
[PMID: 11121513]

[61] Muraoka K, Shimizu K, Sun X, Tani T, Izumi R, Miwa K, *et al.* Flavonoids exert diverse inhibitory effects on the activation of NF-κB. Transplant Proc 2002; 34: 1335-40.
[http://dx.doi.org/10.1016/S0041-1345(02) 02795-1]

[62] Lee WJ, Shim JY, Zhu BT. Mechanisms for the inhibition of DNA methyltransferases by tea catechins and bioflavonoids. Mol Pharmacol 2005; 68(4): 1018-30.
[http://dx.doi.org/10.1124/mol.104.008367] [PMID: 16037419]

[63] Park HH, Lee S, Son HY, *et al.* Flavonoids inhibit histamine release and expression of proinflammatory cytokines in mast cells. Arch Pharm Res 2008; 31(10): 1303-11.
[http://dx.doi.org/10.1007/s12272-001-2110-5] [PMID: 18958421]

[64] Khajuria A, Gupta A, Garai S, Wakhloo B P. Immunomodulatory effects of two sapogenins 1 and 2 isolated from Luffa cylindrica in Balb/C mice. Bioorg Med Chem Lett 2007; 17: 1608-12.
[http://dx.doi.org/10.1016/j.bmcl.2006. 12.091]

[65] Kim GY, Kim KH, Lee SH, *et al.* Curcumin inhibits immunostimulatory function of dendritic cells: MAPKs and translocation of NF-κ B as potential targets. J Immunol 2005; 174(12): 8116-24.
[http://dx.doi.org/10.4049/jimmunol.174.12.8116] [PMID: 15944320]

[66] Kumar A, Dhawan S, Hardegen NJ, Aggarwal BB. Curcumin (Diferuloylmethane) inhibition of tumor necrosis factor (TNF)-mediated adhesion of monocytes to endothelial cells by suppression of cell surface expression of adhesion molecules and of nuclear factor-kappaB activation. Biochem Pharmacol 1998; 55(6): 775-83.
[http://dx.doi.org/10.1016/S0006-2952(97)00557-1] [PMID: 9586949]

[67] Kumar S, Ahuja V, Sankar MJ, Kumar A, Moss AC. Curcumin for maintenance of remission in ulcerative colitis. Cochrane Database Syst Rev 2012; 10: CD008424.
[http://dx.doi.org/10.1002/14651858.CD008424.pub2] [PMID: 23076948]

[68] Singh S, Aggarwal BB. Activation of transcription factor NF-κ B is suppressed by curcumin (diferuloylmethane). J Biol Chem 1995; 270(42): 24995-5000.
[http://dx.doi.org/10.1074/jbc.270.42.24995] [PMID: 7559628]

[69] Xu YX, Pindolia KR, Janakiraman N, Chapman RA, Gautam SC. Curcumin inhibits IL1 alpha and TNF-alpha induction of AP-1 and NF-kB DNA-binding activity in bone marrow stromal cells. Hematopathol Mol Hematol 1997-1998; 11(1): 49-62.
[PMID: 9439980]

[70] Morsch Y, Wang W, Li M, *et al.* Curcumin exerts its antihypertensive effect by down-regulating the AT1 receptor in vascular smooth muscle cells. Sci Rep 2016; 2016(6): 1-8.

[71] Catanzaro M, Corsini E, Rosini M, Racchi M, Lanni C. Immunomodulators inspired by nature: a review on curcumin and Echinacea. Molecules 2018; 23(11): 1-17.
[http://dx.doi.org/10.3390/molecules23112778] [PMID: 30373170]

[72] Shimizu K, Funamoto M, Sunagawa Y, *et al.* Anti-inflammatory action of curcumin and its use in the treatment of lifestyle-related diseases. Eur Cardiol 2019; 14(2): 117-22.
[http://dx.doi.org/10.15420/ecr.2019.17.2] [PMID: 31360234]

[73] Hadi A, Pourmasoumi M, Ghaedi E, Sahebkar A. The effect of Curcumin/Turmeric on blood pressure modulation: A systematic review and meta-analysis. Pharmacol Res 2019; 150: 104505.
[http://dx.doi.org/10.1016/j.phrs.2019.104505] [PMID: 31647981]

[74]   Allam G. Immunomodulatory effects of curcumin treatment on murine schistosomiasis mansoni. Immunobiology 2009; 214(8): 712-27.
[http://dx.doi.org/10.1016/j.imbio.2008.11.017] [PMID: 19249123]

CHAPTER 5

Diagnostic Measures for COVID-19: Current Status and Advances

Aditya Narvekar[1], Darsh Vithlani[3,‡], Ameya Chaudhari[4,‡], Ratnesh Jain[2,*] and Prajakta Dandekar[1,*]

[1] *Department of Pharmaceutical Sciences and Technology, Institute of Chemical Technology, Mumbai-400019, India*

[2] *Department of Chemical Engineering, Institute of Chemical Technology, Mumbai-400019, India*

[3] *Department of Dyestuff Technology, Institute of Chemical Technology, Mumbai-400019, India*

[4] *Department of Biomedical Engineering, Duke University, Durham, North Carolina-27708, USA*

Abstract: The outbreak of COVID-19 in China and its gradual spread over the entire globe, irrespective of age, sex or origin, has posed a major threat to the health of the entire human population. Investigations subsequent to the virus outbreak revealed that the unknown etiology was a novel coronavirus, later referred to as the severe acute respiratory syndrome coronavirus 2 (SARS-CoV-2). The treatment and survival of patients have been largely dependent on an accurate diagnosis of this infection, both in symptomatic and asymptomatic individuals. Thus, highly sensitive and specific laboratory diagnostic methods are imperative for the accurate diagnosis of this condition. This manuscript focuses on various molecular and diagnostic imaging tools for reliable diagnosis of COVID-19 and the correlation of their outcomes with those from previous coronavirus epidemics. The molecular diagnostic tools include real-time reverse transcription polymerase chain reaction (rRT-PCR), ELISA based detection of early humoral response and DNA sequencing. The manuscript will also focus on national and international policies of testing, additional developments, issues and challenges faced in the diagnosis of COVID-19. The chapter will, therefore, highlight the current regime followed, developments and the probable lacunae that, if overcome, could improve the diagnostic schema of this disease.

Keywords: COVID-19, CRISPR, CT scan, Diagnosis, ELISA, FELUDA, Oximetry, RT-LAMP, RT-PCR, SARS-CoV-2, SHERLOCK.

---

* **Corresponding authors Prajakta Dandekar and Ratnesh Jain:** Department of Chemical Engineering, Institute of Chemical Technology, Mumbai-400019, India; Tel: +91-22-3361-2221, Fax: +91-22-3361-10205; and Department of Pharmaceutical Sciences and Technology, Institute of Chemical Technology, Mumbai-400019, India; Tel: +91-22-3361-2029, Fax: +91-22-3361-1020; E-mails: pd.jain@ictmumbai.edu.in and rd.jain@ictmumbai. edu.in
‡ Equal contribution

Jean-Marc Sabatier (Ed.)

INTRODUCTION

The sudden upsurge of coronavirus disease-19 (COVID-19), which originated in Wuhan, China, has engulfed several countries across the globe. It is a global health concern that causes severe respiratory tract infection in humans, as declared by the World Health Organization (WHO). As of August 2020, there were 25 million cases of COVID-19 in several countries across the world, of which 16.4 million cases had recovered, while 0.85 million patients had succumbed to the disease-associated fatalities. The illegal sale of wild animals in the Huanan Seafood Wholesale Market and human consumption of these animal species has been speculated for causing the transmission of severe acute respiratory syndrome coronavirus 2 (SARS-CoV-2) which eventually resulted in the devastating outbreak of COVID-19. Subsequent investigations revealed that a considerable section of the population diagnosed with COVID-19 was not directly linked to this source, indicating person-to-person transmission [1].

SARS-CoV-2 belongs to the family of viruses called Coronaviridae, which possess a single-strand, positive sense RNA genome of approximately 26-32 kilobases. The viral hosts of this family include birds and mammals. Novel coronaviruses have been identified in the recent past, such as the coronavirus of bat origin that led to fatal acute diarrhea syndrome in pigs in 2018 [2]. Coronaviruses, which are pathogenic to humans, usually result in mild clinical symptoms. However, there have been exceptions, such as the severe acute respiratory syndrome coronavirus (SARS-CoV), which originated in Guangdong, southern China, in November 2002. It resulted in 8000 human infections and 774 deaths in 37 countries during 2002-03. The other exception was the Middle East respiratory syndrome coronavirus (MERS-CoV), which was first detected in Saudi Arabia in 2012. It resulted in 2494 laboratory-confirmed infections and 858 deaths as reported in September 2012. Phylogenetic analysis revealed that SARS-CoV-2 shares a sequence identity of approximately 79% with SARS-CoV and approximately 50% with MERS-CoV [3, 4]. Interestingly, SARS-CoV-2 shares a very high sequence identity of approximately 96.3% with the bat coronavirus RaTG13, which was observed in bats from Yunnan in 2013. However, it has been reported that bats are not the immediate source of SARS-CoV-2 [5].

COVID-19 affects different people in different ways. Most infected people are known to develop mild to moderate illness and recover without hospitalization. The most common symptoms of COVID-19 include fever, fatigue, dry cough or dyspnea. The less common symptoms include aches and pains, sore throat, diarrhea, conjunctivitis, headache, loss of taste or smell. After being declared as a pandemic, governments across the world have implemented lockdowns and strict control measures to curb the spread of this disease. Maintaining physical distancing and wearing masks in public are two widely accepted measures that have been observed to control the spread of COVID-19. Despite several preventive measures, cases continue to increase due to the highly contagious nature of this disease and several other factors that are country-specific. The treatment regime for COVID-19 is not specific, and positive cases have been treated using existing anti-viral medicines with an aim to repurpose them. Citizens across the globe are eagerly waiting for a reliable vaccine candidate to be available in the market to obtain relief from the catastrophe caused by this pandemic [1, 6].

Considering the current status of the treatment and vaccination regime for COVID-19, it is very important to follow the sequential strategy of case identification, contact tracing, isolation and testing using a very specific and sensitive laboratory diagnostic technique, as also followed during previous epidemics of SARS-CoV and MERS [7]. In India, several cities have followed the well-known COVID-19 management strategy of 3Ts – testing, tracing and treatment. Considering the population of India, it is difficult to test every individual. However, it cannot be an excuse to justify the insufficient testing in majorly affected cities such as Mumbai, India. Even in the absence of rapid testing kits, oximeter readings were monitored to measure oxygen saturation in densely populated areas such as Dharavi, Mumbai, while massive door-to-door thermal screenings were done in Bengaluru, India. Apart from these strategies, institutional quarantine, stringent containment, use of data analytics for future predictions, regular updates on smartphones through mobile applications such as *Aarogya Setu* and online training and protocols for healthcare workers have been part of the COVID-19 management strategy in India.

It is not practical to use viral cultures for establishing an acute diagnosis of SARS-CoV-2 as it takes a minimum of three days to cause cytopathic effects in cell cultures and also requires biosafety level-3 facilities, which are not available at many healthcare institutions. Considering these drawbacks, reverse transcription-polymerase chain reaction (RT-PCR) has been employed for an accurate laboratory diagnosis of COVID-19 worldwide. The complete genome of SARS-CoV-2 was available early in the epidemic, which facilitated the development of specific primers and standardized laboratory protocols for COVID-19. Several serum antibody-antigen detection-based diagnostic tests are also being developed for quick diagnosis of COVID-19 [8 - 10]. This chapter discusses various diagnostic methods available for COVID-19, including PCR and ELISA based molecular assays. The issues and challenges in the accurate diagnosis of COVID-19 have also been discussed, along with the advancements in this area. The patent summary of COVID-19 diagnostics has also been covered. The chapter will, thus, discuss the complete scenario of COVID-19 diagnosis.

NEED FOR RELIABLE DIAGNOSTIC TOOLS

Reliable diagnosis of any disease dictates the further course of treatment implementation. It is, therefore, of paramount significance to have a reliable diagnostic tool which may influence the fate of the patient inflicted with a disease. It is desirable to have a diagnostic test that is both sensitive as well as specific. However, this is usually a challenging task as increasing sensitivity leads to a decrease in specificity. Hence, depending on the requirement of a particular condition, diagnostic tests are usually designed to achieve a balance between these two factors. Highly sensitive tests are preferred during the early phase of disease diagnosis as they are rarely negative, while highly specific tests are preferred for confirming the diagnosis suggested by the preliminary tests as they are rarely positive. The tests used for preliminary and confirmatory diagnosis should be such that they indicate similar results even through repetitive measurements. There are several factors that are crucial for getting reliable results reproducibly. The principle of the test, the methodology and technical skill are the factors which may affect the test results. These variables, as depicted in Fig. (**1**), must be taken into consideration for a reliable diagnostic test [11 - 13].

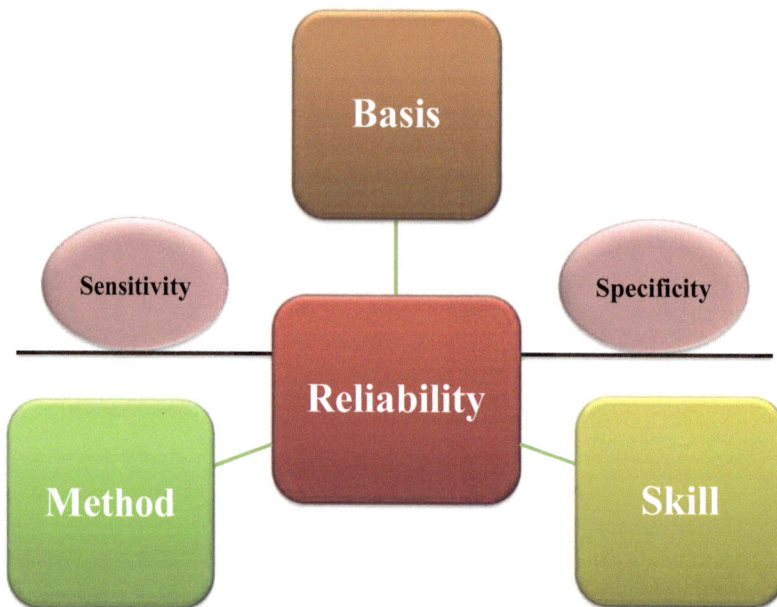

Fig. (1). Factors governing reliability of the diagnostic test.

DIAGNOSTIC METHODS FOR COVID-19

Molecular Assays for Diagnosis of COVID-19

Diagnostic molecular assays generate data related to the presence and concentration of a biological molecule in the sample to be analyzed. The current methods that have been most popularly recommended for diagnosis of COVID-19 by the Center for Disease Control and Prevention (CDC) are the CDC Influenza SARS-CoV-2 Multiplex Assay and the CDC 2019-nCoV RT-PCR Diagnostic Panel, both of which are based on Reverse Transcription-Polymerase Chain Reaction. However, this is not the only technique that may be employed to detect the virus. This document also discusses the other advancements in the field of diagnostics for COVID-19 [14].

CDC Influenza SARS-CoV-2 Multiplex Assay

CDC Influenza SARS-CoV-2 Multiplex Assay test recommended by the CDC is a real-time test, which allows sensitive detection of patient samples in the acute phase of infection. This test was granted emergency use authorization on July 2, 2020. It is real-time RT-PCR or quantitative RT-PCR test which means that the test can monitor the amplification of DNA while the PCR process is ongoing. This test is capable of detecting and differentiating the RNAs from SARS-CoV-2, influenza A virus and influenza B virus at the same time. This test thus allows surveillance of Influenza along with SARS-CoV-2. It will, therefore, aid in management of detection and treatment of COVID-19 by allowing conservation of testing materials and processing upto three times more tests as compared to existing tests for SARS-CoV-2. Human specimens can be taken from the upper or lower respiratory tract. This assay utilizes primers that target the SARS-CoV-2 virus nucleocapsid (N) gene, the influenza A virus matrix (M1) gene and influenza B virus non-structural 2 (NS2) gene. A primer that targets the RNase P gene (RP) for the detection of human nucleic acid is employed as it serves as an internal positive control. These primers are able to amplify the viral genome to yield detectable concentrations. A fluorescent read-out can be used to detect the presence of the virus. The fluorescent read-out is achieved by the addition of specific probes which hybridize with the genomic DNA of the virus. Each cycle leads to the cleavage of additional reporter dye molecules from the probes, increasing the fluorescence intensity. The multiplex assay consists of positive, negative and extraction controls to ensure assay integrity and enables fair comparison of patient samples with the controls. The specimen is considered positive when one or more viral targets cross the threshold before 40.00 Ct. A single specimen may show the presence of multiple viruses. The specimen is considered negative when one or more viral targets cycle threshold curves do not cross the threshold before 40.00 Ct and the RP control crosses the threshold line before 35.00 Ct. When no viral target curve crosses the threshold line before 40.00 Ct, and before 35.00 Ct for RP, then the result is invalid. These results are valid when the controls show expected results, as shown in Table **1** [14].

Table 1. **Result and Interpretation of controls for multiplex assay test.**

Control	Purpose	Influenza A	Influenza B	SARS-CoV-2	RP	Expected Ct
Positive	Extraction and RT-PCR reagent integrity	+	+	+	+	<40.0 for viral genes <35.0 for RP
Negative	Contamination of reagents and environmental contamination	-	-	-	-	None detected ≥40.0 for viral genes ≥35.0 for RP
Extraction	Extraction reagent integrity and contamination	-	-	-	+	<35.0

CDC 2019-nCoV RT-PCR Diagnostic Panel

Another diagnostic method recommended by the CDC is the 2019-nCoV RT-PCR diagnostic panel [15]. This is also a real-time diagnostic technique that was developed by the CDC in early 2020. The kit contains four reagents, namely the primer-probe against the 2019-nCoV_N1, which is the virus nucleocapsid (N) gene, the 2019-nCoV_N2, which is another virus nucleocapsid (N) gene, and the control RP gene for detecting human nucleic acid. Finally, it has nCoVPC as the positive control, which is included in all the panels. This test was given the emergency use authorization on February 4, 2020, by the USFDA. In order to address the global shortage of reagents and materials in diagnostic kits, the USFDA granted an amendment which provided alternatives for performing the test. Additional extraction reagents, extraction instrument and a new process which can be used when there is a shortage of materials were a part of this amendment. The preliminary tests can be conducted by collecting the upper respiratory tract specimens, such as the nasopharyngeal /oropharyngeal (throat) swab, the nasal mid-turbinate (NMT) swab, also called deep nasal swab or nasopharyngeal wash/aspirate or nasal wash/aspirate (NW) specimen. However, a recent report has suggested that sputum specimens give a higher number of true positives in the diagnosis of 2019-nCoV than those from throat swabs [16]. The 2019-nCoV RT-PCR diagnostic panel also consists of positive, negative and extraction controls, as shown in Table **2**. The specimen is considered negative when all viral targets do not cross the threshold before 40.00 Ct, and RP control does cross the threshold line before 35.00 Ct. The specimen is considered positive when all viral targets cross the threshold before 40.00 Ct. The specimen is considered invalid if the viral targets and the RP control markers do not cross the threshold before 40.00 Ct. The result is inconclusive if only one of the viral targets crosses the threshold before 40.00 Ct. Even though RT-PCR is a very robust method, some reports have claimed otherwise. Ren and the group have claimed that there are high number of false negative results due to the thermal inactivation of the samples having a low viral load, which complicates the detection of early stage COVID-19 [17].

Table 2. Result and Interpretation of controls for a diagnostic panel test.

Control	Purpose	N1	N2	RP	Expected Ct
Positive	Extraction and RT-PCR reagent integrity	+	+	+	<40.0
Negative	Contamination of reagents and environmental contamination	-	-	-	None detected
Extraction	Extraction reagent integrity and contamination	-	-	+	<40.0

Enzyme-Linked Immunosorbent Assay (ELISA)

This is a technique used for the detection and quantification of peptides, proteins, antibodies and hormones [18]. The types of ELISA assays used in the diagnosis of COVID-19 are depicted in Fig. (**2**). In the case of indirect ELISA, the antigen is first immobilized on a 96 well plate. The unoccupied sites in the wells are blocked by a blocking agent, such as bovine serum albumin (BSA) or milk protein, to ensure that any non-specific interactions are eliminated. The antibody against the target antigen is then added. Excess unbound antibody is washed away using a suitable buffer. The antibody added for the detection of the target antigen is usually tagged with an enzyme that can convert a chromogenic substrate into a colored end-product, which can be quantified using a UV spectrophotometer. On the other hand, sandwich ELISA involves immobilization of the capture antibody followed by the addition of antigen and detection antibody. The enzyme tagged on the detection antibody can aid quantification of the chromogenic substrate as described previously.

CDC recommends a serologic test using ELISA. Serologic test can be done to detect antibodies against SARS-CoV-2. It is able to identify patients who have been exposed to the SARS-CoV-2 virus prior to analysis. However, this test may not be applicable at an early stage since it requires sufficient stimulation of the immune system to elicit a response against the infectious agent. The test employs a perfusion-stabilized form of the spike protein as a target protein for the detection

[19, 20]. Goat anti-human pan IgG was used as the secondary antibody to improve the specificity and sensitivity of the assay. Although this method resulted in some cross-reactivity with SARS-CoV and MERS-CoV, nonetheless, a specificity greater than 99% and a sensitivity greater than 96% were achieved. The results are interpreted on the basis of the absorbance readings, compared to the positive and negative controls. If the measured absorbance is less than the negative control, the results are reported as negative. Whereas if the measured absorbance is equal to or greater than the positive control, the results are reported as positive. If the measured absorbance is between the negative and positive controls, it is required to re-test the sample, along with other clinical tests. Some tests are detected on the basis of specimen index ratio. The specimen index ratio is calculated using the formula specimen absorbance divided by the cut-off value provided by the manufacturer. If the specimen index ratio is < 1, the result is negative, and if it is ≥ 1, then the result is positive.

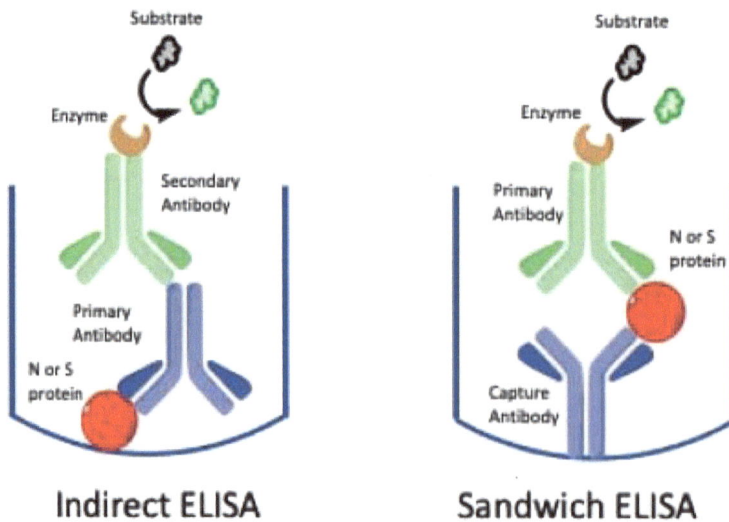

Fig. (2). Types of ELISA used in COVID-19 diagnosis.

Further research in this method led to promising results with the development of recombinant N and S proteins of SARS-CoV-2 for the serological detection of IgG and IgM antibodies. These proteins exhibited reduced cross-reactivity with the other coronaviruses but also yielded consistent results with the nucleic acid detection assay [21]. Another assay protocol employed the SARS-CoV-2S1 protein, expressed in CHO cells, for capturing the antibodies against the virus. This protocol resulted in a specificity of 97.5% and a sensitivity of 97.1% [22]. Researchers have reported the success of serological testing in identifying RT-

PCR-negative, asymptomatic COVID-19 patients. This was attributed to the transient viral shedding duration, which leads to a false negative result during RT-PCR [23]. It has also been proposed that a combination of serological testing and RT-PCR may aid in accurate diagnosis and timely treatment of COVID-19 patients [24].

Antigen Testing

Unlike serological tests in which the human antibodies against the virus are tested, viral antigens can also be detected using an immunoassay. It is based on the same principle as that of ELISA. However, in the case of antigen testing, the antibodies against the viral antigen are used to detect the viral load in the sample. This method is not as popular as the RT-PCR due to its low sensitivity. However, it is less expensive and can be used as a point-of-care diagnostic method since it can detect the virus in as low as 15 min. The CDC has recommended the use of rapid antigen tests for screening in high-risk congregate settings, wherein repeated testing can be quickly performed to identify infected people and avoid transmission. Till now, four emergency use authorizations (EUA) have been given to the rapid antigen tests, where BD and Abbott have manufactured two out of the four tests [25]. The results are interpreted similarly to ELISA-based antibody detection, based on absorbance readings. Even though these EUA have been granted, reports have suggested that rapid antigen testing should not be used as a front-line test method because of its low sensitivity and because the test works well only in cases with high viral loads [26 - 28]. These reports have employed COVID-19 Ag Respi-Strip (Coris Bioconcept, Gembloux, Belgium) as one of the assay kits [26].

DNA Sequencing

The most common method of sequencing is called Sanger Sequencing. In this technique, the DNA sample is added to a mixture of primer, DNA polymerase, and ordinary DNA nucleotides (dATP, dTTP, dGTP, and dCTP). Thereafter, four dye labeled chain-terminating dideoxy nucleotides are added to the reaction mixtures [29]. PCR is performed using a thermocycler in which the DNA polymerase adds nucleotides until the chain-terminating dideoxy nucleotide is added, which terminates the elongation process. The process is repeated a number of times to ensure that each DNA strand ends with a DNA labeled dideoxy nucleotide. Therefore, each DNA strand will have a different chain length with the difference of one nucleotide. These DNA strands will thus be able to reveal the position of each nucleotide in the DNA sample. Sequencing plays a little role in directly diagnosing patients with COVID-19 but plays a huge role in sequencing the genome of COVID-19 so that better diagnostics and therapeutics can be designed against COVID-19. CDC developed its real-time RT-PCR pathogen detection assay based on the genome sequence of the virus [4].

NATIONAL AND INTERNATIONAL POLICIES ON COVID-19 TESTING

The surveillance in India started as early as January 2020 for screening individuals showing symptoms of COVID-19. Several travel advisories and restrictions were issued and Indian nationals arriving from abroad were quarantined. The serious drawback in COVID-19 management in India was the low testing rate considering the population. In order to overcome this flaw, the number of labs was increased from 14 to more than 1596 over the period of 5 months. The testing rate was also increased by the use of rapid antigen and antibody tests along with other molecular diagnostic tests, which remain the gold standard for COVID-19 diagnosis. Several other steps were taken to increase the testing capacity, which included augmentation of testing capacity, upscaling the testing by establishment of mentor institutes, scientific and technical institution upliftment, funding technological innovations for expanding outreach, boosting testing capacity by collaboration with the private sector, setting up quality control processes for quality assurance, putting up validation centers for ensuring quality diagnostic kits, the establishment of a strong supply chain, setting up advisories on diagnostic platforms and forming a partnership to deliver laboratory supplies [30].

The Indian Council of Medical Research (ICMR) along with the Ministry of Health and Family Welfare (MoHFW) undertook the task of expanding the scale of testing by using key approaches such as technology landscaping, leveraging resources and optimization of processes. The government is continuously working on evolving the testing strategy as the country is being reopened in phases. The testing strategy has been expanded and diversified by the use of automated PCR and RNA extraction platforms. The testing capacity was further ramped up by the launch of three high throughput COVID-19 testing facilities. Local vendors and manufacturers are provided government support for the production of materials required for testing under the vision of "Atmanirbhar Bharat" (self-reliant India), thus providing economic upliftment [31].

The policies set out by the European Centre for Disease Prevention and Control (ECDC) aim to achieve several public health objectives based on epidemiological situations. Depending on the pattern of infection in different countries of the European Union, mass testing, targeted testing and/or specific population testing have been carried out. The objective-driven implementation of COVID-19 testing strategies has helped the ECDC to control the pandemic efficiently. The main objectives under COVID-19 testing include monitoring transmission rate and severity of infection, regular testing of health and social care workers, detection of hotspots for mass testing to curb the spread of infection, immediate testing upon symptom onset by providing easy access to testing centers. The testing should be such that it is flexible and adaptable to change depending on the local population dynamics. The re-introduction of infection can be minimized by targeted testing and regular follow-up of individuals from other areas of the same country or from countries where the infection rate is high [32].

ISSUES AND CHALLENGES IN DIAGNOSIS OF COVID-19

RT-PCR has been found to play a pivotal role in the diagnosis of COVID-19. The salient features of the method are its high sensitivity and specificity. However, this method is associated with some limitations. Firstly, the sampling procedure for RT-PCR requires trained personnel so that the swab is taken in a correct manner to minimize the possibility of false-negative results. Also, there is a probability that the viral load present in the respiratory tract at the time of sampling may be insufficient for detection. The detection can be done by analyzing the presence of viral RNA in the bronchoalveolar lavage fluid (BALF). However, this involves the use of suction tools which require experienced handling and can cause discomfort to the patient. False-negative results may also be a consequence of mutations in the primers and regions of the target gene in the genome of the novel coronavirus. Amplification inhibitors present in the sample could also lead to a misleading diagnosis. Molecular targets, such as the genes encoding various structural and accessory genes, have been used for viral load identification. It is important to select an appropriate molecular target as each has a different specificity and sensitivity. If one of the molecular targets yields a positive outcome while the other results in a negative outcome, then the test is inconclusive, and a repeat test is recommended. The primary reason for false-positive results is the contamination of the samples. In RT-PCR, cautious collection, storage and transportation of the sample are extremely essential. Malfunctioning of the instrument, viral recombination and manual errors are amongst the other reasons for erroneous results of RT-PCR. A combination of a nasal and oral swab has been suggested for testing with better accuracy. However, there may be a paucity of swabs or PPE. In such cases, the patients are advised to self-collect the saliva or sputum samples, which could probably lead to ineffective handling of the samples [33 - 40].

The SARS Cov-2 infection begins in the lungs and not in the upper respiratory tract. This, at times, may lead to the lack of compliance between the findings of CT and the results of RT-PCR. During the initial and late stages of COVID-19 infection, the viral load may be too low to enable accurate detection, thus leading to false-negative outcomes. Further, as CT scanning may expose the patients to a potentially harmful dose of radiation, it cannot be used for mass testing. The radiographic features observed in the CT scans of lung cancer patients could indicate COVID-19 associated pneumonia even if the patient has not been actually infected by the virus. In such cases, RT-PCR-based testing has been recommended to confirm the findings of CT to prudently decide upon the therapy to be administered further [41]. Further, the equipment used for CT is expensive and requires trained operators. Moreover, the elaborate sanitation protocols increase the turnover time. Further, to minimize in-hospital cross-contamination, maintenance of a separate ward and a separate hospital staff with personal protection equipment for CT scanning has rendered this method a little expensive. The ground glass opacities, consolidation and some other features of CT could also be imaged *via* CXRs. CXR could also be used in developing countries, having heavy population densities, as a replacement for CT. However, the sensitivity of CXR is only about 69%. It should be noted that detection by CXR is not very effective in the initial stages of the disease. The haziness in the CXR could be misinterpreted as overlying parenchymal tissue or be confused with asthma or some other bacterial pneumonia. Now, the interpretations of CXR are being improved by the use of artificial intelligence and deep learning. This may enable the detection of even the mildest symptoms at early stages, thus enhancing the disease diagnosis [33, 39, 42, 43].

Serodiagnostic methods are regarded as promising tools as they could be implemented on a larger scale for the screening of asymptomatic patients. The immunoglobulin proteins IgG and IgM develop as antibodies to SARS-Cov-infection and are detected around the fourth day after the onset of symptoms. The sensitivity of serodiagnosis by IgM was 77.3%, while that by IgG was 83.3%. They were effectively detected by ELISA in the middle and later stages of the disease. However, the false-negative results have not been eliminated in these investigations. If the concentration of the antibody was below the limit of detection, this method did not work. Particularly, the specific IgG antibodies could take weeks to develop, while the IgM antibodies usually last only for two weeks and are non-specific, making it difficult to diagnose and interpret when the patient is infected. A combination of IgG and IgM serodiagnosis has been, thus, recommended. Another drawback of these methods is their interindividual variability. Although they provide some hints regarding the protocols to be followed subsequently, they cannot be implemented to confirm the presence of the virus. The Deep Sequencing methods have been used to observe the mutations in the SARS-Cov-2 and they are not a viable method for diagnosing the infection in patients [34, 40, 44]. A compendious overview of the widely used methods for the diagnosis of SARS-Cov-2 has been shown in Table **3**.

Table 3. Overview of diagnostic methods and initial screening of COVID-19 [45 - 52].

Method of Diagnosis	Sensitivity and Specificity	Time Required	Possible Reasons for a False Positive	Possible Reasons for a False Negative	Other Disadvantages	Advantages
RT-PCR	High sensitivity and specificity, low limit of detection	2-4 hours	1. Contamination while sampling 2. Manual errors and malfunctioning of the instrument	1. Inappropriate sampling procedure 2. Mutations in the primers and regions of the target gene 3. Amplification inhibitors present in the sample	1. Prone to pre-analytical, analytical and post-analytical errors 2. Long turn over time 3. Not economically viable for mass testing in most developing nations	1. The accuracy of this method is a striking advantage
Serodiagnosis	Commendable specificity and sensitivity	15-30 minutes	1. Patients with high levels of rheumatoid factor or HAMA antibodies 2. Cross coupling	1. Level of antibodies below the limit of detection 2. Antibodies assayed not yet developed	1. The immune response varies from one individual to another 2. No information obtained about the inception of the virus	1. Can be implemented for mass testing 2. Economic
Computed Tomography (CT)	High sensitivity but moderate specificity which can be improved upon by AI	30 minutes	1. Features could indicate viral pneumonia due to some other virus videlicet; adenovirus 2. Erroneous interpretation of radiographic features observed in the ct scans of lung cancer patients	1. Misdiagnosis as a common infection	1. Patients exposed to harmful radiation 2. Elaborate sanitation procedures to be followed in the CT ward	1. Accuracy comparable to that of RT-PCR, infact ct may show abnormalities even if the RT-PCR is negative 2. Severity of the infection can be gauged.

(Table 3) cont.....

Method of Diagnosis	Sensitivity and Specificity	Time Required	Possible Reasons for a False Positive	Possible Reasons for a False Negative	Other Disadvantages	Advantages
Chest X-Ray (CXR)	High sensitivity and specificity achieved with the use of deep learning based convoluted neural networks	15 minutes	1. Faulty interpretation of the features	1. Haziness in the CXR misinterpreted as overlying parenchymal tissue or confused with asthma or some other bacterial pneumonia 2. Features are usually not that evident during the onset of the disease	1. Exposure to radiation 2. The CXR usually does not show any abnormalities in the early stages of the infection	1. Relieved the load of CT 2. Easier to perform in isolated wards without the elaborate sanitation procedures as required in CT 3. Can be a useful technique if the patient cannot move 4. More economic

Apart from the issues and challenges specific to COVID-19 diagnosis, several issues which are common to the diagnosis of all diseases also apply to the diagnosis of COVID-19. Several common errors such as sample misidentification, inappropriate collection, unsuitable transportation and storage may lead to erroneous results. Experimental, technical and instrumental errors may also significantly jeopardize the quality of testing and should be regularly validated before commencing the diagnosis [39, 53]. COVID-19 has questioned our expertise, technological advancements, preparedness and the ability of even the developed nations to handle and control the pandemic. It is of utmost importance to be cognizant of the various pre-analytical, analytical and post-analytical errors possible during diagnosis. The diagnostic methods play a cardinal role in containing the spread of the virus for tracing the infected persons and initiating the available treatments. However, the drawbacks need to be addressed by paying a significant amount of attention to developing robust diagnostic methods [53 - 55].

ADVANCEMENTS IN DIAGNOSTIC TOOLS FOR COVID-19

The conventional diagnostic techniques for COVID-19, which have been approved by the WHO, have been discussed in Section 3. PCR, ELISA and sequencing methods play a crucial role in routine clinical diagnosis and discovery of novel strains of bacteria, viruses and other pathogens. These techniques have therefore been specified in the WHO guidelines for clinical diagnosis of COVID-19 [56]. However, these methods are time-consuming and cause a delay in the diagnosis and treatment. This has exposed the shortcomings of the existing diagnostic methods and clinical testing infrastructure, which is extremely essential in such health emergencies. On a positive note, COVID-19 has helped to speed up the R & D efforts to develop simple, rapid, cost-effective and sensitive diagnostic methods [57]. Various modified diagnostic methods, such as nested rRT-PCR, RT-PCR with locked nucleic acid probes and RT-loop mediated isothermal amplification have been reported for the detection of COVID-19. Nested rRT-PCR combines two rounds of PCR amplification with real-time detection approach, thus providing an alternative and sensitive method for the detection of COVID-19. Findings by Jiang *et al.* revealed that real time nested PCR exhibited several advantages over the conventional methods. It was simple and rapid to perform and did not require strenuous processing steps involved in nested and/or RT-PCR. The crucial steps which involved demanding RT procedures, such as the use of regular thermocycler for nested PCR and use of agarose gels were bypassed, and thus, test results could be obtained within 4-5 h. This dual real-time PCR method could be easily completed within 2 h using LightCycler. It involved a 45-min, one-step RT-PCR, followed by 40-min real-time nested PCR, making it an ideal routine protocol for high-throughput screening of SARS-CoV-containing samples. This assay had a detection limit of <10 copies of SARS-CoV, which reduced the number of false-negative results for samples containing the only minor viral load. The developed assay was sensitive enough to detect trace amounts of virus in the sample, suggesting that this test was an excellent alternative to the existing assay methods for SARS-CoV, which frequently generated false-negative results for samples collected during the early phase of infection. The results from the assay were interpreted on the basis of fluorescence-based amplification of the viral DNA from the samples [58]. Another modification of PCR that has been favourably utilized is the RT-PCR with locked nucleic acid (LNA) probes. Several single nucleotide mismatches have been reported in the primers and probes in the existing assays, which has affected the assay sensitivity. Chan *et al.* hypothesized that additional gene targets may be suitable for designing RT-PCR for CoVs and would increase the options for molecular diagnosis of circulating and emerging CoV infections. LNA probes-based novel real-time RT-PCR assays have been designed by researchers through the identification of abundantly expressed leader sequence in the 5'-untranslated region (UTR) in small-RNA-Seq data analysis for clinically important CoVs. Small-RNA-Seq data analysis was used for the determination of the most abundantly expressed sequences in the CoV genome. It was hypothesized that an abundantly present leader sequence might be a beneficial diagnostic target and the infected cells contain large quantity of viral subgenomic RNA. LNA probes were employed to overcome the relatively short length of the leader sequences. LNA is a nucleic acid analogue with an extra bridge connecting the 2' oxygen and 4' carbon that has exceptionally high hybridization affinity towards complementary DNA and RNA and efficient mismatch discrimination. These properties are linked with the increased melting temperature of the oligonucleotides. This allows utilization of shorter probes when LNA rather than DNA nucleotides are used in the nucleic acid amplification assays. Hence, the selection of optimal gene targets by utilizing small-RNA-Seq data analysis for the development of molecular diagnostic assays and the previously unknown diagnostic value of the CoV leader sequence was demonstrated through this study. Probes were labeled at the 5' end, with the reporter molecule 6-carboxyfluorescein, and the results were interpreted on the basis of an increase in fluorescence intensity. The application of LNA probes thus allowed the use of relatively short sequences as a diagnostic target in RT-PCR assays. Development of these assays into multiplex assays, with comparable sensitivity and specificity, and additional detection of other novel or re-emerging CoVs may further enhance their clinical utility [59]. One more variant of PCR, *i.e.* reverse transcription-loop-mediated isothermal amplification (RT-LAMP), is a genetic diagnostic method that has been widely used for the detection of viral pathogens. Shirato *et al.* demonstrated a novel RT-LAMP assay using primer sets targeting a conserved nucleocapsid protein region for the detection of MERS-CoV. The RT-LAMP method required only a single temperature for amplification, which provided the results in less than 1 h by observation of magnesium pyrophosphate precipitate or fluorescence signals by the naked eye. This assay can be performed using basic laboratory equipment, such as a heating block and water bath, although real-time monitoring of the assay can be performed using a turbidimeter. This method has been validated using various respiratory viruses, as well as more diverse pathogens, such as bacteria, protozoa and parasites. Furthermore, the reagents necessary to perform RT-LAMP are commercially available. The RT-LAMP assay is highly sensitive and is capable of detecting as few as 3.4 copies of MERS-CoV RNA, and is highly specific, with no cross-reaction to other respiratory viruses. The assay is interpreted using fluorescent signals, under ultraviolet light, following completion of the amplification reaction. Green fluorescent light is considered as a signal of successful amplification. The sensitivity of RT-LAMP assay is similar to that of MERS-CoV real-time RT-PCR. The RT-LAMP assay is, therefore, a useful tool and can be further extrapolated for the diagnosis and epidemiologic surveillance of several other CoV infections [60]. On a similar trajectory, a one-step, one-tube assay based on real-time RT-PCR was developed by Dharavath *et al.* with automated analysis for detection of SARS-CoV-2. A combination detection method was designed in which a novel primer targeted SARS-CoV-2 Nucleocapsid N gene sequence with two primer pairs. Each pair probed with another non-overlapping region of SARS-CoV-2 Nucleocapsid N gene and ORF1ab gene, respectively. SYBR Green I and Taqman probes have been used in qRT-PCR based detection of SARS-CoV-2. SYBR Green-based qRT-PCR protocol is comparatively economical but the non-specific binding of the dye to DNA compromises the specificity and sensitivity of the assay, with the limit of detection of 150 copies of viral RNA molecules/reaction. TaqMan probe-based protocol has a higher sensitivity and can detect as low as 15 copies of viral RNA molecules/reaction. It is a multiplex assay based on two virus-specific target probes, which are fluorescently labeled. It is a single tube, one step qRT-PCR reaction. Therefore, the assay fulfills WHO guidelines on the reliability of results, wherein at least two genomic targets are required for a diagnostic test. The results are based on fluorescence detection of labeled dual TaqMan test probes with 6-FAM (6-Carboxyfluorescein)/BHQ-1 (Black hole quencher-1), which target the unique regions of the SARS-CoV-2 *Nucleocapsid* gene along with an internal reference control gene *RNase P* probe, labeled with HEX-1 (Hexachloro fluorescein-1) / BHQ-1, simultaneously. The data generated from this RT-PCR assay was quantitatively assessed by a graphical user interface, COVID qPCR Analyzer, a tool for reproducible down-stream analysis and automated report generation of the analyses samples. There are several shortcomings of this method with respect to sequence alignment, method accuracy and variability and, therefore, require further validation using a large number of samples [61].

CRISPR-based detection of COVID-19 with isothermal amplification has been developed and can be used for the detection of RNA viruses. Zhang *et al.* have developed a CRISPR-based SHERLOCK (Specific High Sensitivity Enzymatic Reporter UnLOCKing) technique for the detection of COVID-19. They have been able to consistently detect COVID-19 target sequences, in a range between 10-100 copies/microliter of input, using synthetic COVID-19 virus RNA fragments. The test can be carried out using RNA purified from patient samples and can be read out using a dipstick, in less than an hour, without the requirement of elaborate instrumentation. The protocol involves three steps and can be completed in 1 h, from nucleic acid extraction till the qRT-PCR step. The first step involves isothermal amplification of the extracted nucleic acid sample, using a commercially available recombinase polymerase amplification (RPA) kit, during an incubation period of 25 min. The pre-amplified viral RNA sequence is detected using Cas13 in the second step, having an incubation period of 30 min. The final step includes a visual readout of the detection result, using a commercially-available paper dipstick and an incubation period of 2 min [62]. Another CRISPR-based detection method incorporates Cas9 ortholog from *Francisella novicida* (FnCas9) that shows a very high mismatch sensitivity under *in vitro* and *in vivo* conditions. It is distinct from the engineered Cas proteins but shows similar specificity. It shows negligible binding affinity to substrates that harbor mismatches. Azhar *et al.* have reasoned that FnCas9 mediates DNA interrogation and subsequent cleavage. This property can be adapted for accurately identifying any single nucleotide variants, provided that the fundamental mechanism of discrimination is consistent across all sequences. This approach has been named FnCas9 Editor Linked Uniform Detection Assay (FELUDA). FELUDA couples sensitivity with a broad spectrum of read-out possibilities, which can be carried out in the lab or in the field owing to the highly specific binding and subsequent cleavage properties of FnCas9. The results from FELUDA can be precisely determined using agarose or capillary electrophoresis. It can be adapted as a fluorescence-based readout, which is widely used for several CRISPRDx platforms. FELUDA is also capable of providing a highly accurate diagnosis of single nucleotide variants, and thus, detection of low copy numbers is easier and does not require the use of additional molecules on CRISPR platforms. It, therefore, shows utility in various pathological conditions, including genetic disorders and infectious diseases such as COVID-19 [63]. The advancements in the diagnosis methods for COVID-19 have been comprehensively depicted in Fig. (**3**).

Apart from developments of quick confirmatory tests, there is also a need for early identification of COVID-19. Currently, diagnostic tests are recommended for those showing symptoms of the disease, but that may not be sufficient for delaying the transmission rate of the virus. Raman spectroscopy has been reported to detect biomarkers of several viral diseases and can prove as a potential technique for carrying out mass testing. Wyllie *et al.* have described a comparable sensitivity of SARS-CoV-2 detection in the saliva of an asymptomatic COVID-19 patient. Thus, the USFDA has approved a saliva-based diagnostic kit. Saliva offers a quick and non-invasive alternative to nasopharyngeal swabs for detecting SARS-CoV-2. Desai *et al.* have developed a novel statistical model for the detection of RNA viruses in saliva. It is based on an unbiased selection of a set of 65 Raman spectral features that mostly attribute to the RNA moieties. They have also developed a GUI-based analytical tool "RNA Virus Detector (RVD)" to minimize variability and to automate the downstream analysis of the Raman spectra. This conceptual framework to detect RNA viruses from saliva would aid in the application of Raman Spectroscopy for managing viral outbreaks, such as the ongoing COVID-19 pandemic [64].

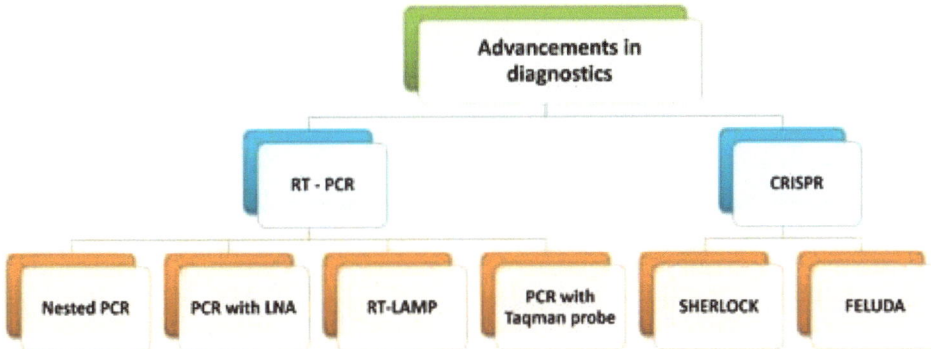

Fig. (3). Overview of advancements in COVID-19 diagnosis.

PATENT SCENARIO OF COVID-19 DIAGNOSTICS

The declaration of COVID-19 public health emergency on February 4, 2020 has led to the development of about 100 molecular diagnostic tests of SARS-CoV-2 under emergency use authorization by the FDA. Several tests have been developed for the management of COVID-19, which include thirty-seven molecular laboratory- tests, two antigen diagnostic tests, twenty-five serology/antibody tests and one *in vitro* diagnostic test. The previous research and innovation in the area of COVID-19 diagnostics have aided in the development of diagnostic tests for emergency use during the COVID-19 pandemic as it is not the first time exposure to this fatal infection. The number of patents published and patent applications on the diagnosis of SARS-CoV were used as a useful barometer to assess innovation to fight SARS-CoV. Previous patents and patent publications on the diagnosis of SARS-CoV suggest that previous SARS-CoV outbreaks stimulated innovation related to the diagnosis of COVID-19 [65].

10,326 patent publications were identified in a systemic worldwide search of patent databases for coronavirus or severe acute respiratory syndrome coronavirus. These were divided into 2,652 simple patent application families. 599 publications were from the United States alone among these 2652 publications. Table **4** shows the largest Intellectual Property Offices with the breakdown of the patent applications [66].

Table 4. Number of patent applications from different countries.

Countries	Number of Applications
WIPO	240
China	616

(Table 4) cont.....

Countries	Number of Applications
Europe	189
Japan	179
South Korea	169
United States	599

New measures were implemented by The United States Patent and Trademark Office (USPTO) in order to hasten innovations related to COVID-19. The voluntary licensing and commercialization of innovations in the area of COVID-19 was prioritized by the USPTO. They also launched the Patents 4 Partnerships IP marketplace platform to facilitate the same. The number of published patents is likely to spike in 16 to 18 months from the initial outbreak, with the governments across the world supporting research and innovations. It is hoped that these patents provide a feasible solution to the eradication, treatment and early diagnosis of this disease and benefit mankind [67].

CONCLUSION

Previously developed technologies which took decades for development and process optimization have played a crucial role in the diagnosis of disease. Researchers have been able to design COVID-19 diagnostics with the aid of the available diagnostic technologies. Experience with previous epidemics, such as SARS and MERS, has been found to be instrumental in the development of COVID-19 identification and detection. The widespread havoc created due to the pandemic has compelled the development of quicker diagnostic methods in order to prevent the further spread of the disease. The current method of infra-red thermal scanning of the forehead cannot detect asymptomatic or pre-symptomatic patients, nor can it distinguish COVID-19 infection from other respiratory illnesses. RT-PCR diagnostic method has greater sensitivity and specificity but requires several hours for detection. Rapid antibody-based diagnostic tests are not specific and may not be suitable for mass testing. This has compelled the development of diagnostic tools that are rapid as well as sensitive. Diagnostic methods, such as RT-LAMP, CRISPR based SHERLOCK and FELUDA, *etc.* give promising results in less time, and thus, need to be deployed immediately after regulatory approval. Several of these promising diagnostic tools have been developed as point-of-care devices in order to overcome the limitations of testing in remote areas. Many of these are in various stages of approval and are expected to be used by laboratories soon. These developments in the area of diagnostics would aid in the advancement of diagnostics for other disease conditions as well. The area of COVID-19 diagnosis is greatly evolving and new information is being updated daily. Many studies reported in this chapter are associated with their own drawbacks and thus, require attention, while some studies referred are preprints, which have not been peer-reviewed. It is, thus, important to note that many of the upcoming diagnostics may not translate to patient use given the stringent guidelines for regulatory approval.

CONSENT FOR PUBLICATION

Not applicable.

CONFLICT OF INTEREST

The authors confirm that this chapter contents have no conflict of interest.

ACKNOWLEDGEMENTS

A.N. is thankful to DST-India for Inspire Fellowship (IF170661). The corresponding authors are thankful to the Ramanujan fellowship research grant (SR/S2/RJN -139/2011) and Ramalingaswami fellowship research grant (BT/RLF/Re-entry/51/2011) for financial support towards generating lab infrastructure. The authors are thankful to Ms. Pankti Ganatra for providing the Chest X-ray and CT scan report of a COVID-19 positive patient.

LIST OF ABBREVIATIONS

SARS-CoV-2	Severe acute respiratory syndrome coronavirus 2
COVID-19	Coronavirus disease-19
MERS	Middle East respiratory syndrome
rRT-PCR	Real-Time Reverse Transcription Polymerase Chain Reaction
CT	Computed Tomography
WHO	World Health Organization
R & D	Research and development
ORF	Open Reading Frame Proteins
ARDS	Acute Respiratory Distress Syndrome
SaO$_2$	Arterial Oxygen Partial Pressure
LEDs	Light Emitting Diodes
SpO2	oxygen saturation by pulse oximetry
PBA	Probe Based Applications
CBA	Camera Based Applications
CXR	Chest X-Rays

GGO	Ground glass opacities
BALF	Broncho alveolar lavage fluid
LNA	Locked nucleic acid
UTR	Untranslated region
RT-LAMP	Reverse transcription-loop-mediated isothermal amplification
GUI	Graphical user interface
CRISPR	Clustered regularly interspaced short palindromic repeats
SHERLOCK	Specific High Sensitivity Enzymatic Reporter UnLOCKing
FELUDA	FnCas9 Editor Linked Uniform Detection Assay
RPA	Recombinase polymerase amplification
RVD	RNA Virus Detector
FDA	Food and drug administration
USPTO	United States Patent and Trademark Office
CDC	Center for Disease Control and Prevention
Taq	Thermus aquaticus
N gene	Nucleocapsid gene
ELISA	Enzyme-Linked Immunosorbent Assay
CHO	Chinese Hamster Ovary
EUA	Emergency use authorization
NMT swab	Nasal mid-turbinate swab
RP gene	RNase P gene
NS2 gene	Non-structural 2 gene
Ct	Cycle threshold
HAMA	Human anti-mouse antibodies

REFERENCES

[1]   Zhai P, Ding Y, Wu X, Long J, Zhong Y, Li Y. The epidemiology, diagnosis and treatment of COVID-19. Int J Antimicrob Agents 2020; 55(5)105955
[http://dx.doi.org/10.1016/j.ijantimicag.2020.105955] [PMID: 32234468]

[2]   Su S, Wong G, Shi W, *et al.* Epidemiology, genetic recombination, and pathogenesis of coronaviruses. Trends Microbiol 2016; 24(6): 490-502.
[http://dx.doi.org/10.1016/j.tim.2016.03.003] [PMID: 27012512]

[3]   Zhu N, Zhang D, Wang W, *et al.* China Novel Coronavirus Investigating and Research Team. A novel coronavirus from patients with pneumonia in China, 2019. N Engl J Med 2020; 382(8): 727-33.
[http://dx.doi.org/10.1056/NEJMoa2001017] [PMID: 31978945]

[4]   Lu R, Zhao X, Li J, *et al.* Genomic characterisation and epidemiology of 2019 novel coronavirus: implications for virus origins and receptor binding. Lancet 2020; 395(10224): 565-74.
[http://dx.doi.org/10.1016/S0140-6736(20)30251-8] [PMID: 32007145]

[5]   Zhou P, Fan H, Lan T, *et al.* Fatal swine acute diarrhoea syndrome caused by an HKU2-related coronavirus of bat origin. Nature 2018; 556(7700): 255-8.
[http://dx.doi.org/10.1038/s41586-018-0010-9] [PMID: 29618817]

[6]   Xie X, *et al.* Chest CT for typical 2019-nCoV pneumonia: relationship to negative RT-PCR testing. Radiology 2020; 200343-3.

[7]   Zhou P, *et al.* A pneumonia outbreak associated with a new coronavirus of probable bat origin. Nature 2020; 579(7798): 270-3.

[8]   Peiris JS, Lai ST, Poon LL, *et al.* SARS study group. Coronavirus as a possible cause of severe acute respiratory syndrome. Lancet 2003; 361(9366): 1319-25.
[http://dx.doi.org/10.1016/S0140-6736(03)13077-2] [PMID: 12711465]

[9]   Chana JF-W, Yip C, To K. Improved molecular diagnosis of COVID-19 by the novel, highly sensitive and specific 2 COVID-19-RdRp/Hel realtime reverse transcription-polymerase chain reaction assay validated 3 *in vitro* and with clinical specimens. J Clin Microbiol 2020; 00310-20.

[10]   Chan JF-W, Kok KH, Zhu Z, *et al.* Genomic characterization of the 2019 novel human-pathogenic coronavirus isolated from a patient with atypical pneumonia after visiting Wuhan. Emerg Microbes Infect 2020; 9(1): 221-36.
[http://dx.doi.org/10.1080/22221751.2020.1719902] [PMID: 31987001]

[11]   Kyriacou DN. Reliability and validity of diagnostic tests. Acad Emerg Med 2001; 8(4): 404-5.
[http://dx.doi.org/10.1111/j.1553-2712.2001.tb02125.x] [PMID: 11282682]

[12]   Greenland S. Introduction to stratified analysis. In: Rothman K, Greenland S, Eds. Modern Epidemiology 1998; 253-79.

[13]   Fletcher R, Fletcher S, Wagner E. Cause Clinical Epidemiology. 3rd ed. Baltimore: Lippincott Williams & Wilkins 1996; pp. 228-48.

[14]   CDC. CDC Diagnostic Tests for COVID-19 2020.

[15]   CDC. CDC's Diagnostic Test for COVID-19 Only and Supplies 2020.

[16]   Lin C, Xiang J, Yan M, Li H, Huang S, Shen C. Comparison of throat swabs and sputum specimens for viral nucleic acid detection in 52 cases of novel coronavirus (SARS-Cov-2)-infected pneumonia (COVID-19). Clin Chem Lab Med 2020; 58(7): 1089-94.
[http://dx.doi.org/10.1515/cclm-2020-0187] [PMID: 32301745]

[17]   Pan Y, Long L, Zhang D, *et al.* Potential false-negative nucleic acid testing results for Severe Acute Respiratory Syndrome Coronavirus 2 from thermal inactivation of samples with low viral loads. Clin Chem 2020; 66(6): 794-801.
[http://dx.doi.org/10.1093/clinchem/hvaa091] [PMID: 32246822]

[18]   Alhajj M, Farhana A. Enzyme Linked Immunosorbent Assay (ELISA), in StatPearls. StatPearls Publishing 2020.

[19]   Wrapp D, Wang N, Corbett KS, *et al.* Cryo-EM structure of the 2019-nCoV spike in the prefusion conformation. Science 2020; 367(6483): 1260-3.
[http://dx.doi.org/10.1126/science.abb2507] [PMID: 32075877]

[20]   Freeman B, Lester S, Mills L, *et al.* Validation of a SARS-CoV-2 spike protein ELISA for use in contact investigations and serosurveillance. bioRxiv 2020.2020.04.24.057323
[PMID: 32511332]

[21]   Zhong L, Chuan J, Gong B, *et al.* Detection of serum IgM and IgG for COVID-19 diagnosis. Sci China Life Sci 2020; 63(5): 777-80.
[http://dx.doi.org/10.1007/s11427-020-1688-9] [PMID: 32270436]

[22]   Zhao R, *et al.* Early detection of SARS-CoV-2 antibodies in COVID-19 patients as a serologic marker of infection. Clin Infect Dis 2020.

[23]   Wu J, Liu X, Zhou D, *et al.* Identification of RT-PCR-Negative asymptomatic COVID-19 patients *via* serological testing. Front Public Health 2020; 8: 267.
[http://dx.doi.org/10.3389/fpubh.2020.00267] [PMID: 32582617]

[24]   Wang P. Combination of serological total antibody and RT-PCR test for detection of SARS-COV-2 infections. J Virol Methods 2020; 283113919
[http://dx.doi.org/10.1016/j.jviromet.2020.113919] [PMID: 32554043]

[25]   USFDA. *In Vitro* Diagnostics EUAs. 2020.

[26]   Scohy A, Anantharajah A, Bodéus M, Kabamba-Mukadi B, Verroken A, Rodriguez-Villalobos H. Low performance of rapid antigen detection test as frontline testing for COVID-19 diagnosis. J Clin Virol 2020; 129104455
[http://dx.doi.org/10.1016/j.jcv.2020.104455] [PMID: 32485618]

[27]   Mak GC, Cheng PK, Lau SS, *et al.* Evaluation of rapid antigen test for detection of SARS-CoV-2 virus. J Clin Virol 2020; 129104500
[http://dx.doi.org/10.1016/j.jcv.2020.104500] [PMID: 32585619]

[28]   Ikeda M, *et al.* Clinical evaluation of self-collected saliva by RT-qPCR, direct RT-qPCR, RT-LAMP, and a rapid antigen test to diagnose COVID-19. medRxiv 2020.

[29]   Heather JM, Chain B. The sequence of sequencers: The history of sequencing DNA. Genomics 2016; 107(1): 1-8.
[http://dx.doi.org/10.1016/j.ygeno.2015.11.003] [PMID: 26554401]

[30]   ASIA, N.. India's COVID-19 arc slows as daily testing capacity hits 1.5m. 2020. Available from: https://asia.nikkei.com/Spotlight/Coronavirus/India-s-COVID-19-arc-slows-as-daily-testing-capacity-hits-1.5m

[31]   WHO-India. How India scaled up its laboratory testing capacity for COVID19 2020. Available from: https://www.who.int/india/news/feature-stories/detail/how-india-scaled-up-its-laboratory--esting-capacity-for-covid19

[32]   Control ECDPa. COVID-19 testing strategies and objectives Technical report. 2020. Available from: https://www.ecdc.europa.eu/en/publications-data/covid-19-testing-strategies-and-objectives#no-link

[33]   Chen S-G, Chen JY, Yang YP, Chien CS, Wang ML, Lin LT. Use of radiographic features in COVID-19 diagnosis: Challenges and perspectives. J Chin Med Assoc 2020; 83(7): 644-7.
[http://dx.doi.org/10.1097/JCMA.0000000000000336] [PMID: 32349032]

[34]   Xiang F, *et al.* Antibody detection and dynamic characteristics in patients with COVID-19. Clin Infect Dis 2020.

[35]   Phan T. Genetic diversity and evolution of SARS-CoV-2. Infect Genet Evol 2020; 81104260
[http://dx.doi.org/10.1016/j.meegid.2020.104260] [PMID: 32092483]

[36]   Al-Sadi AM, Al-Oweisi FA, Edwards SG, Al-Nadabi H, Al-Fahdi AM. Genetic analysis reveals diversity and genetic relationship among Trichoderma isolates from potting media, cultivated soil and uncultivated soil. BMC Microbiol 2015; 15(1): 147.
[http://dx.doi.org/10.1186/s12866-015-0483-8] [PMID: 26215423]

[37]   Wang Y, Zhang L, Sang L, *et al.* Kinetics of viral load and antibody response in relation to COVID-19 severity. J Clin Invest 2020; 130(10): 5235-44.
[http://dx.doi.org/10.1172/JCI138759] [PMID: 32634129]

[38]   Tahamtan A, Ardebili A. Real-time RT-PCR in COVID-19 detection: issues affecting the results. Taylor & Francis 2020.

[39]   Lippi G, Simundic A-M, Plebani M. Potential preanalytical and analytical vulnerabilities in the laboratory diagnosis of coronavirus disease 2019 (COVID-19). Clin Chem Lab Med 2020; 58(7): 1070-6.
[http://dx.doi.org/10.1515/cclm-2020-0285] [PMID: 32172228]

[40] Tang Y-W, Schmitz JE, Persing DH, Stratton CW. Laboratory diagnosis of COVID-19: current issues and challenges. J Clin Microbiol 2020; 58(6)e00512-20
[http://dx.doi.org/10.1128/JCM.00512-20] [PMID: 32245835]

[41] Allegra A, Pioggia G, Tonacci A, Musolino C, Gangemi S. Cancer and SARS-CoV-2 Infection: Diagnostic and Therapeutic Challenges. Cancers (Basel) 2020; 12(6): 1581.
[http://dx.doi.org/10.3390/cancers12061581] [PMID: 32549297]

[42] Wong HYF, *et al.* Frequency and distribution of chest radiographic findings in COVID-19 positive patients. Radiology 2020.201160
[PMID: 32216717]

[43] Vickers NJ. Animal communication: when i'm calling you, will you answer too? Curr Biol 2017; 27(14): R713-5.
[http://dx.doi.org/10.1016/j.cub.2017.05.064] [PMID: 28743020]

[44] Li Z, Yi Y, Luo X, *et al.* Development and clinical application of a rapid IgM-IgG combined antibody test for SARS-CoV-2 infection diagnosis. J Med Virol 2020; 92(9): 1518-24.
[http://dx.doi.org/10.1002/jmv.25727] [PMID: 32104917]

[45] Schiaffino S, Tritella S, Cozzi A, *et al.* Diagnostic performance of chest x-ray for COVID-19 pneumonia during the SARS-CoV-2 pandemic in Lombardy, Italy. J Thorac Imaging 2020; 35(4): W105-6.
[http://dx.doi.org/10.1097/RTI.0000000000000533] [PMID: 32404797]

[46] Minaee S, *et al.* Deep-covid: Predicting covid-19 from chest x-ray images using deep transfer learning. arXiv preprint arXiv 2020; 09363.

[47] Kim H, Hong H, Yoon SH. Diagnostic performance of CT and reverse transcriptase-polymerase chain reaction for coronavirus disease 2019: a meta-analysis. Radiology 2020; 296(3): E145-55.
[http://dx.doi.org/10.1148/radiol.2020201343] [PMID: 32301646]

[48] Lebedin YS, *et al.* The Importance of SARS-CoV-2 N-Ag serodiagnostics for the management of covid-19 pneumonia in hospital settings 2020.

[49] Li Y, Xia L. Coronavirus disease 2019 (COVID-19): role of chest CT in diagnosis and management. AJR Am J Roentgenol 2020; 214(6): 1280-6.
[http://dx.doi.org/10.2214/AJR.20.22954] [PMID: 32130038]

[50] Alizad-Rahvar AR, *et al.* False-negative mitigation in group testing for COVID-19 screening. medRxiv 2020.

[51] Yamaoka Y, Jeremiah SS, Miyakawa K, *et al.* Whole nucleocapsid protein of SARS-CoV-2 may cause false positive results in serological assays. Clin Infect Dis 2020.ciaa637
[http://dx.doi.org/10.1093/cid/ciaa637] [PMID: 32445559]

[52] Cardiology ESo. Diagnostic Imaging in COVID-19 2020.

[53] Younes N, Al-Sadeq DW, Al-Jighefee H, *et al.* Challenges in Laboratory Diagnosis of the Novel Coronavirus SARS-CoV-2. Challenges in Laboratory Diagnosis of the Novel Coronavirus SARS-CoV-2. Viruses 2020; 12(6): 582.
[http://dx.doi.org/10.3390/v12060582] [PMID: 32466458]

[54] Hope Michael D, *et al.* A role for CT in COVID-19? What data really tell us so far. http://www. thelancet. com/article/S0140673620307285/pdf2020.

[55] van Zyl G, Maritz J, Newman H, Preiser W. Lessons in diagnostic virology: expected and unexpected sources of error. Rev Med Virol 2019; 29(4)e2052
[PMID: 31145511]

[56] Kumar R, Nagpal S, Kaushik S, Mendiratta S. COVID-19 diagnostic approaches: different roads to the same destination. Virusdisease 2020; 31(2): 97-105.
[http://dx.doi.org/10.1007/s13337-020-00599-7] [PMID: 32656306]

[57]   Sheridan C. COVID-19 spurs wave of innovative diagnostics. Nat Biotechnol 2020; 38(7): 769-72.
[http://dx.doi.org/10.1038/s41587-020-0597-x] [PMID: 32641849]

[58]   Jiang SS, Chen TC, Yang JY, *et al*. Sensitive and quantitative detection of severe acute respiratory syndrome coronavirus infection by real-time nested polymerase chain reaction. Clin Infect Dis 2004; 38(2): 293-6.
[http://dx.doi.org/10.1086/380841] [PMID: 14699465]

[59]   Chan JF-W, Choi GK, Tsang AK, *et al*. Development and evaluation of novel real-time reverse transcription-PCR assays with locked nucleic acid probes targeting leader sequences of human-pathogenic coronaviruses. J Clin Microbiol 2015; 53(8): 2722-6.
[http://dx.doi.org/10.1128/JCM.01224-15] [PMID: 26019210]

[60]   Shirato K, Yano T, Senba S, *et al*. Detection of Middle East respiratory syndrome coronavirus using reverse transcription loop-mediated isothermal amplification (RT-LAMP). Virol J 2014; 11(1): 139.
[http://dx.doi.org/10.1186/1743-422X-11-139] [PMID: 25103205]

[61]   Dharavath B, Yadav N, Desai S, *et al*. A one-step, one-tube real-time RT-PCR based assay with an automated analysis for detection of SARS-CoV-2. Heliyon 2020; 6(7)e04405
[http://dx.doi.org/10.1016/j.heliyon.2020.e04405] [PMID: 32665985]

[62]   Kellner MJ, Koob JG, Gootenberg JS, Abudayyeh OO, Zhang F. SHERLOCK: nucleic acid detection with CRISPR nucleases. Nat Protoc 2019; 14(10): 2986-3012.
[http://dx.doi.org/10.1038/s41596-019-0210-2] [PMID: 31548639]

[63]   Azhar M, *et al*. Rapid, field-deployable nucleobase detection and identification using FnCas9. bioRxiv 2020.

[64]   Desai S, Mishra SV, Joshi A, *et al*. Raman spectroscopy-based detection of RNA viruses in saliva: A preliminary report. J Biophotonics 2020; 13(10)e202000189
[http://dx.doi.org/10.1002/jbio.202000189] [PMID: 32609429]

[65]   USFDA. Emergency Use Authorization 2020.

[66]   Peden AS. AFK, Coronavirus Innovation Guideposts on the Eve of the COVID-19 Pandemic 2020.

[67]   Brinckerhoff CC. New Platform to Facilitate Development of COVID-19 Technologies 2020.

CHAPTER 6

Herd Immunity: An Indirect Protection Against COVID-19

Prashant Tiwari[1,*] and **Pratap Kumar Sahu**[2]

[1] *School of Pharmacy, Arka Jain University, Jamshedpur, Jharkhand, India*

[2] *School of Pharmaceutical Sciences, Siksha O Anusandhan Deemed to be University, Bhuba-neswar, Odisha, India-751029*

Abstract: COVID-19 is an infectious as well as contagious disease caused by severe acute respiratory syndrome (SARS) - Cov2 virus. As of date there is no specific treatment for coronavirus infection. Only symptomatic treatment is given to corona positive patients. Herd immunity is a natural phenomenon providing indirect protection against infectious diseases that are contagious. The principle behind herd immunity is that if enough immune persons are present in a community, then that will interrupt the transmission of an infectious agent and provide indirect protection for susceptible or unimmunized individuals. There are two ways to achieve herd immunity, either by mass vaccination or by allowing the disease to make its round through the population. Since vaccine development is a time taking process, herd immunity can be achieved by unleashing the virus in a controlled way. Sweden is the world leader of herd immunity in the fight against the corona virus. However, there are limitations to using herd immunity worldwide to stop the spread of this novel corona virus.

Keywords: COVID-19, Herd immunity, Vaccination.

INTRODUCTION

Immunity is the defense mechanism of our body against any pathogen or invading agent. The study of immunity is called immunology. There are 3 lines of defense. The first line is the physical barrier which includes the surface barriers like intact skin, mucous membrane, tear, saliva, urine and other body fluids [1, 2]. The second line of response is the non-specific response against any pathogen. The third line of defense is the specific immune response to a variety of pathogens in a specific manner. This specific immune response is adapted or acquired when the first two lines are inadequate [3, 4].

* **Corresponding author Prashant Tiwari:** School of Pharmacy, Arka Jain University, Jamshedpur, Jharkhand, India; Tel: +91-7828865022; E-mail:dr.prashant@arkajainuniversity.ac.in

Jean-Marc Sabatier (Ed.)

Immunity can be innate or acquired. Innate immunity is due to an individual's constitutional make up. It is a non-immunological response. Negroes are resistant to yellow fever than whites because of innate immunity [5, 6]. When the innate immunity is inadequate, acquired immunity develops. Acquired immunity can either be active or passive. Both active and passive immunity can either be naturally acquired or artificially stimulated [7, 8]. Types of immunity are shown in Fig. (**1**).

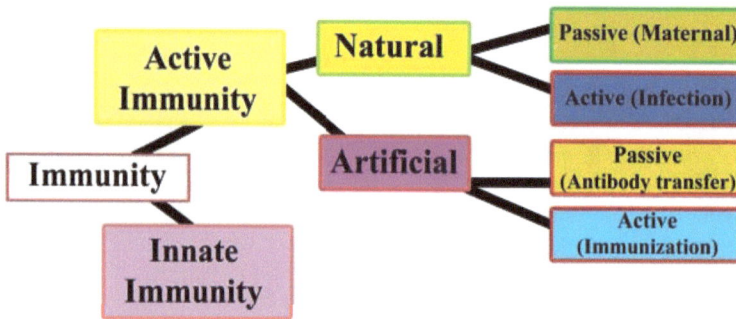

Fig (1). Types of immunity.

Antigen is the foreign substance when introduced into the body that can produce disease. Our body in response to antigen produces antibodies. The antibodies can eliminate antigens to make us free from diseases [9, 10]. In the first exposure to antigen, the body recognizes the antigen and subsequently produces antibodies specific to the antigen. The production of antibodies is a time taking process. So, there is every chance of disease in the first exposure itself if enough load of the pathogen is introduced into the body. During the second exposure, the antibodies are already there, so they can eliminate the antigen [11, 12].

Following a clinical infection, a person naturally acquires immunity as antibodies are developed against the pathogen. So, the person never suffers from the disease for the second time if he suffers from the disease like polio, diphtheria *etc* [13]. During a sub-clinical infection (the person is exposed to the pathogen without any symptoms), the pathogen load is not enough to produce the disease but can protect the person during second exposure because of presence of antibodies [14]. Immunity developed after clinical or sub-clinical infection is called active immunity as the immune system is in action mode after the exposure of antigen to produce antibody. Naturally the fetus obtains the antibodies from its mother which can protect the fetus up to 6 months after birth. This is called passive immunity [15].

Both active and passive immunities can also be acquired or stimulated artificially. The live attenuated (toxoid) or killed (suspensions of microorganisms) form of the pathogen (antigen) can be administered to induce the production of antibodies [16]. These preparations are called as vaccines. Passive immunity can be produced artificially by directly injecting antibodies produced in an animal like horse, sheep, ox, rabbit, *etc* [17]. The antigen or venom is injected into the healthy animal to induce production of antibodies in the animal. When a satisfactory degree of immunity is produced, a large volume of blood is withdrawn from the animal and serum is separated [18]. This serum now contains the antibody (immunoglobulin) or the anti-venom or anti-toxin and accordingly the preparations are known as sera or anti-sera [19]. In emergency cases of infections with novel infectious agents, since the antibody preparations are not developed, the convalescent plasma containing antibodies from individuals who have recovered from that novel infection can be administered [20 - 22].

The antigen containing preparations (vaccines) can stimulate active immunity. The immunity develops slowly but has a lasting effect. They are used for long term prophylaxis. The antibody containing preparations (sera and anti-sera) can stimulate passive immunity. The immunity provided is immediate but temporary. They are used for therapeutic purpose and short-term prophylaxis [23, 24]. Vaccination of children has protected them from many diseases which were once the major cause of morbidity and mortality [25, 26]. The World Health Organization (WHO) and the governments of different countries are encouraging and facilitating mass immunisation through planned vaccination programmes [27].

When a large percentage of individuals in a population or community are immunized against an infection either through mass immunization or post infection, then they provide protection to those persons who are not immune. In this condition, we say the population has developed herd immunity [28, 29]. COVID-19 is a pandemic caused by severe acute respiratory syndrome (SARS) - Cov2 virus. Since there is neither specific treatment nor vaccines for corona virus infection, herd immunity can be achieved through infections only by allowing the infection to run through the population in a controlled way.

HERD IMMUNITY

Herd immunity is also known as herd effect or community immunity or population immunity or social immunity. In herd immunity, all individuals in the population are not immune. A certain percentage of the population is only immune. Immune persons act as a barrier for the non-immune persons and protect them against the infection. When herd immunity is achieved, the population will become resistant to the infection. There will be no spreading of the disease from one person to another and the outbreak will stop [30 - 32]. So, herd immunity provides indirect protection from the disease. Herd immunity is crucial for those individuals who cannot become immune due to medical reasons like immuno-suppression or immuno-deficiency [33, 34].

Herd immunity was first recognized as a naturally occurring phenomenon in the 1930s when the number of cases of measles reduced due to immunity among a significant number of children infected with measles [35, 36]. However, this was temporary. It was the measles vaccine which helped in achieving herd immunity. Mass vaccination using measles vaccine in 1960s controlled and almost eliminated measles. But the communities with inadequate vaccination help the measles virus return to those communities [37 - 39].

Herd immunity has some success stories against few illnesses. People in Norway successfully developed herd immunity (though partial) against swine flu (H1N1 virus) through vaccination and natural immunity [40, 41]. Small pox was eradicated from the world in 1977 due to herd immunity achieved through effective vaccination [42]. Measles and chickenpox were very common among children, but the use of vaccines developed herd immunity and these diseases are now extremely rare in developed countries like the United States [43, 44].

Herd immunity has reduced the frequency of many diseases, if not eliminate them. Use of meningococcal sero group C conjugate (MCC) vaccines developed herd immunity and reduced the number of cases significantly in unimmunized individuals [45]. Similarly, oral cholera vaccines quickly protect a population for a period of time. However, the protection depends on vaccine efficacy, vaccine coverage, and the rate of mobility of the population [46]. In Scotland, a national human papillomavirus (HPV) immunization program significantly lowered the HPV infection among nonvaccinated women within 5 years' time from 2008 to 2013 [47]. India is doing a mass vaccination campaign to control and eventually eradicate foot-and-mouth disease (FMD) [48].

PRINCIPLE OF HERD IMMUNITY

The principle underlying herd immunity is that the presence of enough persons in a community immune to the disease interrupts the transmission of the disease, thereby providing indirect protection to susceptible or un-immunized individuals [49 - 52]. There will be a reduced probability of an un-immunized individual becoming infected when he is part of an immunized or vaccinated population (Fig. 2). This can be explained by a term called herd immunity threshold (HIT). It represents a certain percentage of population who, when become immune to a certain disease, can eliminate that disease from the population [53]. It is not necessary that 100% of a population need to become immune to eradicate a disease. HIT varies from disease to disease and is given in Table **1**. It may vary from 40% (for H1N1) to 94% (for measles) [54 - 56].

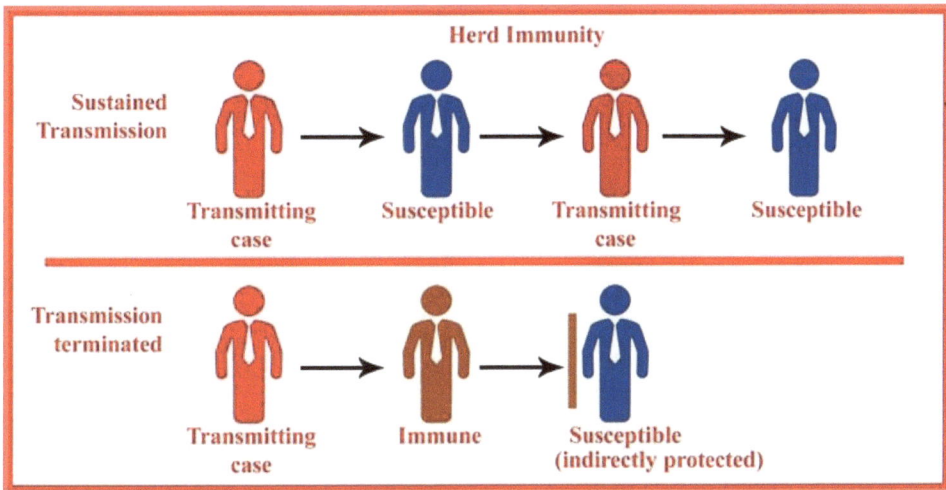

Fig (2). Principle of herd immunity.

Table 1. Herd immunity threshold (HIT) for different infectious and contagious diseases.

Disease	Herd Immunity Threshold (HIT)
Small pox	83-85%
Measles	83-94%
Mumps	75-86%
Rubella	83-85%
Diphtheria	85%
Pertussis	92-94%
Polio	80-86%
Pandemic flu (H1N1)	~40%
COVID-19	60-80%

When immunity develops in a population and certain threshold (HIT) is reached, there will be gradual elimination of the disease from that population. The disease will be eradicated when HIT is reached worldwide [57]. Herd immunity is not applicable to all infectious diseases. It is only applicable to those infectious diseases which are contagious (spreads from person to person) [58]. Tetanus is an infectious disease but not contagious. So, herd immunity is not applicable to tetanus. COVID-19 infectious and also spreads from person to person. So, herd immunity is applicable to COVID-19 [59, 60].

DEVELOPING HERD IMMUNITY

There are 2 ways to produce herd immunity against a disease:

1. Develop and administer a safe and effective vaccination.
2. Wait for the disease to make its round through a population.

Vaccines provide the attenuated or killed form of the microorganism against which antibodies are developed so that when actual infection occurs these antibodies protect the body against the virus [61 - 63]. Clinical or Sub clinical infection also develops antibodies against the microorganism and the person becomes immune. But clinical infection can be a cause of morbidity and in some cases mortality. Between these two methods, vaccination is the safer method as it is a preventive method [64 - 66].

Advances in vaccine technology could open new opportunities in the control of several infectious diseases [67]. DNA recombinant technologies and nanoscale engineering are revolutionizing the development of vaccines [68, 69]. In recent times vaccination has been found to effectively reduce the incidence of many diseases like influenza [70 - 72], respiratory syncytial virus (RSV) [73], *etc.* Education about herd immunity along with local vaccination coverage can encourage people to vaccinate which will be helpful to both individuals and communities [74]. Opposition to vaccines resistance against vaccinations, financial/logistical challenges and a lack of vaccines that provide long-term protection is the major challenge to herd immunity [75].

COVID-19

Endemic is a term that defines a disease or condition within a specific location. Malaria is endemic to parts of Africa. When the number of endemic cases becomes greater than anticipated, the endemic becomes an outbreak [76 - 78]. If the outbreak is not controlled immediately, then it becomes an epidemic and affects a large number of populations. A pandemic is an epidemic that spreads from one country to another. COVID-19 is a pandemic [79].

Severe acute respiratory syndrome (SARS) - Cov-2 is the virus that causes COVID-19. The virus is new to humans. No one has immunity against it. So, virus spreads quickly and easily. It is observed that 80% of corona positive patients require no treatment [80]. Less than 20% of corona positive patients need hospitalization. A very small proportion of them (mainly with underlying chronic illness) need admission in the intensive care unit (ICU). This disease is known to occur in all age groups. Old persons and persons with pre-existing diseases like blood pressure, heart disease, lungs disease, diabetes, cancer, *etc.* are at relatively high risk and appear to develop serious illness than others [81 - 83].

Our immune system has a major role in treatment or prevention of COVID-19. Once a person is infected, he naturally develops active immunity and there will be presence of antibodies in his blood [84]. Use of vaccines in the form of attenuated virus or killed suspension of the virus can induce active immunity artificially. We can also use antibodies to provide passive immunity [85]. Currently there are no vaccines, monoclonal antibodies (mAbs), or drugs available for SARS-CoV-2. Many vaccines are under clinical trial.

Again, the antibodies in the form of sera are not developed yet. Human convalescent plasma is an option for the prevention and treatment of COVID-19. Convalescent plasma (immunoglobulin-containing serum) is obtained from the blood of people who have recovered and show the willingness to donate. [86, 21]. At least two persons can be benefitted from one donor. Convalescent plasma, when administered to selected patients with severe symptoms, is found to recover them [20].

COVID 19 AND HERD IMMUNITY

COVID 19 is a highly infectious/contagious disease which progressing rapidly throughout the world. The major common symptoms of coronavirus include cold, fever, sore throat, fatigue and adenoids. In severe cases, people may face other symptoms like confusion, blush face or lips, difficulty in waking, high fever, swelling and redness of hands and legs decreased white blood cells, persistent chest pain, coughing up blood, kidney failure and finally death. Complications of COVID 19 may lead to acute respiratory distress, pneumonia, sepsis and kidney failure. Keeping in view of its severity, it needs to be controlled at the earliest. Now we are only controlling its spread through social distancing and the use of sanitizers. But we can completely eradicate it either through vaccines or through clinical or subclinical infection [87, 88].

a. Herd immunity through vaccination:

The vaccines are in development stage undergoing preclinical trials and clinical studies. The list of vaccines and their current status against SARS-Cov-2 is given in Table **2**. However, vaccination has following limitations.

i. There is opposition to vaccination in certain communities.
ii. SARS-Cov-2 is highly mutating. So, vaccine against one strain may not be effective against another mutated strain.

Table 2. List of vaccines under development against COVID-19 and their current status [89].

S.No.	Name of Vaccine	Company and Country	Mechanism	Current Status
1	ZyCoV-D	Zydus Cadila, India	The first approach is DNA vaccination. Second approach is live attenuated recombinant measles virus vectored against COVID 19.	Phase-II
2	Novavax	Serum Institute, India	Enhancing antigen presentation in local lymph nodes, boosting immune responses	Phase-I/ Phase-II
3	No name yet	Biological E, India	-	Phase-I/ Phase-II
4	Covaxin	Bharat Biotech, India	Prevent SARS-CoV-2 coronavirus infections	Phase-I/ Phase-II
5	No name yet	Mynvax, India	-	Phase-I/ Phase-II
6	No name yet	Indian Immunologicals, India	-	Phase-I/ Phase-II
7	Otezla	Amgen and Adaptive Biotechnologies, US	Treating respiratory distress in late-stage patients	Pre-clinical
8	AdCOVID	Altimmune, UK	-	Pre-clinical/Phase-I
9	BNT162	BioNTech and Pfizer, Germany	Prevent SARS-CoV-2 coronavirus infections	Phase-I/ Phase-II
10	Leronlimab	CytoDyn, US	Mild-to-moderate respiratory complications	Phase 2 and Phase 2b/3
11	Remdesivir	Gilead Sciences, US	Interferes with the action of viral RNA-dependent RNA polymerase and evades proofreading by viral exoribonuclease	Phase-III
12	AS03	GlaxoSmithKline, UK	The *mechanism* of action of *AS03* remains unclear	Phase-I/ Phase-II

(Table 2) cont.....

S.No.	Name of Vaccine	Company and Country	Mechanism	Current Status
13	No name yet	Heat Biologics, US	-	Pre-clinical/Phase-I
14	INO-4800	Inovio Pharmaceuticals, US	Strengthening the body's own natural response *mechanisms*	Phase 1 clinical trial
15	Vaccine	Johnson & Johnson, US	Training the immune system to recognize and combat pathogens	Preclinical
16	mRNA-1273	Moderna, US	-	Phase 1
17	NVX-CoV2373	Novavax, US	Predicts induction of functional antibodies that may block infection.	Phase 1
18	REGN-COV2	Regeneron Pharmaceuticals, US	Bind non-competitively to the critical receptor binding domain of the virus's spike protein	Preclinical
19	Kevzara	Regeneron Pharmaceuticals and Sanofi, US	Inhibits IL-6 receptor signaling	Phase 2/3
20	Actemra	Roche, Switzerland	Binds to both soluble and membrane-bound IL-6 receptors	Phase 3
21	No name yet	Sanofi, France	-	Preclinical
22	TAK-888	Takeda Pharmaceutical, Japan	Development of anti-SAR--CoV-2 polyclonal hyperimmune globulin (H-IG)	Preclinical
23	No name yet	Vaxart, US	-	Phase 1
24	VIR-2703, VIR-7831 and VIR-7832	Vir Biotechnology, US	Target the SARS-CoV-2 spike protein and are effective at neutralising the virus in live virus-cellular assays.	Preclinical

b) Herd immunity through clinical or sub clinical infection:

Since vaccines are under development, herd immunity can be achieved if the disease is prevalent in the population. The person who is exposed to the coronavirus will show symptoms (clinical infection) or may be asymptomatic (sub clinical infection) [90, 91]. In both the cases, he develops antibodies against the virus and becomes immune. This process will continue until herd immunity threshold (HIT) is achieved. So this is a time taking process. Again it is a double edged sword as development of immunity is associated with risk of morbidity and mortality [92 - 94]. It must be used judiciously as life of every human being is important. The people who are at high risk like elderly people, immuno-compromised people, people with chronic illness and children should be kept safe and away from the social exposure. However, this will not be an easy task [95, 96].

Sweden is the world champion of herd immunity in the fight against corona virus. It has allowed the virus to spread in a controlled way. Citizens of Sweden practice social distancing on a voluntary basis. The restrictions imposed by Swedish authorities to flatten the curve are not harsh. There were no fines, no policing, no location-tracing technologies and no apps [97, 98].

India is a country of young population with about 93.5% of its population younger than 65. India can take the risk of employing the strategy of herd immunity by allowing the disease to run through the population in a controlled way [99]. People below 60 years of age can be allowed to live normal life with social distancing, masks and hand sanitizers. Herd immunity can be achieved if we let them get infected and recover so that everybody will be immune to the virus [100, 101], but we have to take care of those who are at high risk [30, 102].

Herd immunity achieved through this method has following limitations:

  i. When we allow people to become infected, there may be a sudden increase in number of patients. The COVID hospitals run by the government may not have enough beds. This may increase the number of casualties before herd immunity is reached.
 ii. The number of patients with lifestyle disorders is ever increasing even in young patients. So, mortality may be more than expected.
iii. The herd immunity threshold for COVID-19 is about 60-80% which is at the higher side.
 iv. Different strains of corona virus are existing due to the ability of the virus to mutate. Herd immunity achieved against one strain may allow other existing strain to spread.

CONCLUSION

Use of vaccines is the safest way to achieve herd immunity in a certain population. Allowing the disease to run through the population has many associated risks, especially when we do not have a clear understanding of the disease pathology. People with high risk such as elderly people, children and people with chronic illness may become very sick if exposed to the virus. Many vaccines are under clinical trial. Only time will tell the success of these vaccines against mutating strains of coronavirus. The reason behind severe illness in some patients, whereas mild symptoms in others, should be explored to develop a suitable vaccine.

CONSENT FOR PUBLICATION

Not Applicable.

CONFLICT OF INTEREST

The author confirms that this chapter contents have no conflict of interest.

ACKNOWLEDGEMENTS

The authors are grateful to the Regional Medical Research Centre (RMRC), Bhubaneswar, Odisha, India for providing literature assistance to make this work successful.

REFERENCES

[1]　Daneman R, Rescigno M. The gut immune barrier and the blood-brain barrier: are they so different? Immunity 2009; 31(5): 722-35.
[http://dx.doi.org/10.1016/j.immuni.2009.09.012] [PMID: 19836264]

[2]　Cummings JH, Antoine JM, Azpiroz F, *et al.* PASSCLAIM--gut health and immunity. Eur J Nutr 2004; 43(2) (Suppl. 2): II118-73.
[PMID: 15221356]

[3]　Blanco JL, Garcia ME. Immune response to fungal infections. Vet Immunol Immunopathol 2008; 125(1-2): 47-70.
[http://dx.doi.org/10.1016/j.vetimm.2008.04.020] [PMID: 18565595]

[4]　Whyte SK. The innate immune response of finfish--a review of current knowledge. Fish Shellfish Immunol 2007; 23(6): 1127-51.
[http://dx.doi.org/10.1016/j.fsi.2007.06.005] [PMID: 17980622]

[5]　Kassiotis G, Stoye JP. Immune responses to endogenous retroelements: taking the bad with the good. Nat Rev Immunol 2016; 16(4): 207-19.
[http://dx.doi.org/10.1038/nri.2016.27] [PMID: 27026073]

[6]　Batista-Duharte A, Lindblad EB, Oviedo-Orta E. Progress in understanding adjuvant immunotoxicity mechanisms. Toxicol Lett 2011; 203(2): 97-105.
[http://dx.doi.org/10.1016/j.toxlet.2011.03.001] [PMID: 21392560]

[7]　Baxter D. Active and passive immunity, vaccine types, excipients and licensing. Occup Med (Lond) 2007; 57(8): 552-6.
[http://dx.doi.org/10.1093/occmed/kqm110] [PMID: 18045976]

[8]　Rooke JA, Bland IM. The acquisition of passive immunity in the new-born piglet. Livest Prod Sci 2002; 78(1): 13-23.
[http://dx.doi.org/10.1016/S0301-6226(02)00182-3]

[9]　Warrington R, Watson W, Kim HL, Antonetti FR. An introduction to immunology and immunopathology. Allergy Asthma Clin Immunol 2011; 7(S1) (Suppl. 1): S1.
[http://dx.doi.org/10.1186/1710-1492-7-S1-S1] [PMID: 22165815]

[10] Davies DR, Padlan EA, Sheriff S. Antibody-antigen complexes. Annu Rev Biochem 1990; 59(1): 439-73.
[http://dx.doi.org/10.1146/annurev.bi.59.070190.002255] [PMID: 2197980]

[11] Boyden SV. Natural antibodies and the immune response.Advances in immunology. Academic Press 1966; Vol. 5: pp. 1-28.

[12] Lamm ME. Interaction of antigens and antibodies at mucosal surfaces. Annu Rev Microbiol 1997; 51(1): 311-40.
[http://dx.doi.org/10.1146/annurev.micro.51.1.311] [PMID: 9343353]

[13] Collins FM, Pearsall NN. Cellular antimicrobial immunity. CRC Crit Rev Microbiol 1978; 7(1): 27-91.
[http://dx.doi.org/10.3109/10408417909101177] [PMID: 383406]

[14] Read AF, Mackinnon MJ. Pathogen evolution in a vaccinated world. Evolution in health and disease 2008; 2: 139-52.

[15] Jeffcott LB. Passive immunity and its transfer with special reference to the horse. Biol Rev Camb Philos Soc 1972; 47(4): 439-64.
[http://dx.doi.org/10.1111/j.1469-185X.1972.tb01078.x] [PMID: 4574242]

[16] Stephens JM. Immunity in insects. Insect Pathology 2012; 1: 273-97.

[17] Beveridge WI. Immunity to viruses. Viral and Rickettsial Infections of Animals 1967; 1: 313-3.
[http://dx.doi.org/10.1016/B978-1-4832-3319-2.50014-7]

[18] Leon G, Sanchez L, Hernández A, *et al.* Immune response towards snake venoms. Inflammation & Allergy-Drug Targets (Formerly Current Drug Targets-Inflammation & Allergy) 2011; 10(5): 381-98.
[http://dx.doi.org/10.2174/187152811797200605]

[19] Gazarian KG, Gazarian T, Hernández R, Possani LD. Immunology of scorpion toxins and perspectives for generation of anti-venom vaccines. Vaccine 2005; 23(26): 3357-68.
[http://dx.doi.org/10.1016/j.vaccine.2004.12.027] [PMID: 15837360]

[20] Duan K, Liu B, Li C, *et al.* Effectiveness of convalescent plasma therapy in severe COVID-19 patients. Proc Natl Acad Sci USA 2020; 117(17): 9490-6.
[http://dx.doi.org/10.1073/pnas.2004168117] [PMID: 32253318]

[21] Casadevall A, Pirofski LA. The convalescent sera option for containing COVID-19. J Clin Invest 2020; 130(4): 1545-8.
[http://dx.doi.org/10.1172/JCI138003] [PMID: 32167489]

[22] Shen C, Wang Z, Zhao F, *et al.* Treatment of 5 critically ill patients with COVID-19 with convalescent plasma. JAMA 2020; 323(16): 1582-9.
[http://dx.doi.org/10.1001/jama.2020.4783] [PMID: 32219428]

[23] Bloch EM, Shoham S, Casadevall A, *et al.* Deployment of convalescent plasma for the prevention and treatment of COVID-19. J Clin Invest 2020; 130(6): 2757-65.
[http://dx.doi.org/10.1172/JCI138745] [PMID: 32254064]

[24] Tanne JH. Covid-19: FDA approves use of convalescent plasma to treat critically ill patients. BMJ 2020; 368: m1256.
[http://dx.doi.org/10.1136/bmj.m1256] [PMID: 32217555]

[25] Pollard AJ, Perrett KP, Beverley PC. Maintaining protection against invasive bacteria with protein-polysaccharide conjugate vaccines. Nat Rev Immunol 2009; 9(3): 213-20.
[http://dx.doi.org/10.1038/nri2494] [PMID: 19214194]

[26] Edwards KM. Overview of pertussis: focus on epidemiology, sources of infection, and long term protection after infant vaccination. Pediatr Infect Dis J 2005; 24(6) (Suppl.): S104-8.
[http://dx.doi.org/10.1097/01.inf.0000166154.47013.47] [PMID: 15931137]

[27]   Woodle D. Vaccine procurement and self-sufficiency in developing countries. Health Policy Plan 2000; 15(2): 121-9.
[http://dx.doi.org/10.1093/heapol/15.2.121] [PMID: 10837034]

[28]   Nielsen A, Larsen SO. Epidemiology of pertussis in Denmark: the impact of herd immunity. Int J Epidemiol 1994; 23(6): 1300-8.
[http://dx.doi.org/10.1093/ije/23.6.1300] [PMID: 7721534]

[29]   Fine PE. Herd immunity: history, theory, practice. Epidemiol Rev 1993; 15(2): 265-302.
[http://dx.doi.org/10.1093/oxfordjournals.epirev.a036121] [PMID: 8174658]

[30]   Fine P, Eames K, Heymann DL. "Herd immunity": a rough guide. Clin Infect Dis 2011; 52(7): 911-6.
[http://dx.doi.org/10.1093/cid/cir007] [PMID: 21427399]

[31]   Gonçalves G. Herd immunity: recent uses in vaccine assessment. Expert Rev Vaccines 2008; 7(10): 1493-506.
[http://dx.doi.org/10.1586/14760584.7.10.1493] [PMID: 19053206]

[32]   Kim TH, Johnstone J, Loeb M. Vaccine herd effect. Scand J Infect Dis 2011; 43(9): 683-9.
[http://dx.doi.org/10.3109/00365548.2011.582247] [PMID: 21604922]

[33]   Schneider-Schaulies J. Cellular receptors for viruses: links to tropism and pathogenesis. J Gen Virol 2000; 81(Pt 6): 1413-29.
[http://dx.doi.org/10.1099/0022-1317-81-6-1413] [PMID: 10811925]

[34]   Richens J, Mabey DC. Section System-oriented Disease. Manson's Tropical Diseases 2008; 16: 403.

[35]   Anderson RM, May RM. Vaccination against rubella and measles: quantitative investigations of different policies. J Hyg (Lond) 1983; 90(2): 259-325.
[http://dx.doi.org/10.1017/S002217240002893X] [PMID: 6833747]

[36]   Pyle GF. Measles as an urban health problem: the Akron example. Econ Geogr 1973; 49(4): 344-56.
[http://dx.doi.org/10.2307/143237]

[37]   Strebel PM, Papania MJ, Fiebelkorn AP, Halsey NA. Measles vaccine. Vaccines (Basel) 2012; 6: 352-87.

[38]   Dew K. Epidemics, panic and power: representations of measles and measles vaccines. Health 1999; 3(4): 379-98.
[http://dx.doi.org/10.1177/136345939900300403]

[39]   Nokes DJ, Swinton J. Vaccination in pulses: a strategy for global eradication of measles and polio? Trends Microbiol 1997; 5(1): 14-9.
[http://dx.doi.org/10.1016/S0966-842X(97)81769-6] [PMID: 9025230]

[40]   Lang PO, Aspinall R. Immunosenescence and herd immunity: with an ever-increasing aging population do we need to rethink vaccine schedules? Expert Rev Vaccines 2012; 11(2): 167-76.
[http://dx.doi.org/10.1586/erv.11.187] [PMID: 22309666]

[41]   Lipsitch M, Finelli L, Heffernan RT, Leung GM. Redd; for the 2009 H1N1 Surveillance Group SC. Improving the evidence base for decision making during a pandemic: the example of 2009 influenza A/H1N1. Biosecur Bioterror 2011; 9(2): 89-115.
[PMID: 21612363]

[42]   Anderson RM, May RM. Vaccination and herd immunity to infectious diseases. Nature 1985; 318(6044): 323-9.
[http://dx.doi.org/10.1038/318323a0] [PMID: 3906406]

[43]   Gershon AA. Live-attenuated varicella vaccine. Infect Dis Clin North Am 2001; 15(1): 65-81, viii.
[http://dx.doi.org/10.1016/S0891-5520(05)70268-3] [PMID: 11301823]

[44]   Marin M, Meissner HC, Seward JF. Varicella prevention in the United States: a review of successes and challenges. Pediatrics 2008; 122(3): e744-51.

[http://dx.doi.org/10.1542/peds.2008-0567] [PMID: 18762511]

[45]   Trotter CL, Maiden MC. Meningococcal vaccines and herd immunity: lessons learned from serogroup C conjugate vaccination programs. Expert Rev Vaccines 2009; 8(7): 851-61.
[http://dx.doi.org/10.1586/erv.09.48] [PMID: 19538112]

[46]   Peak CM, Reilly AL, Azman AS, Buckee CO. Prolonging herd immunity to cholera *via* vaccination: Accounting for human mobility and waning vaccine effects. PLoS Negl Trop Dis 2018; 12(2)e0006257
[http://dx.doi.org/10.1371/journal.pntd.0006257] [PMID: 29489815]

[47]   Cameron RL, Kavanagh K, Pan J, *et al.* Human papillomavirus prevalence and herd immunity after introduction of vaccination program, Scotland, 2009–2013. Emerg Infect Dis 2016; 22(1): 56-64.
[http://dx.doi.org/10.3201/eid2201.150736] [PMID: 26692336]

[48]   Singh RK, Sharma GK, Mahajan S, *et al.* Foot-and-Mouth Disease Virus: Immunobiology, Advances in Vaccines and Vaccination Strategies Addressing Vaccine Failures-An Indian Perspective. Vaccines (Basel) 2019; 7(3): 90.
[http://dx.doi.org/10.3390/vaccines7030090] [PMID: 31426368]

[49]   Field RI, Caplan AL. A proposed ethical framework for vaccine mandates: competing values and the case of HPV. Kennedy Inst Ethics J 2008; 18(2): 111-24.
[http://dx.doi.org/10.1353/ken.0.0011] [PMID: 18610781]

[50]   Roeder PL, Taylor WP. Mass vaccination and herd immunity: cattle and buffalo. Rev Sci Tech 2007; 26(1): 253-63.
[http://dx.doi.org/10.20506/rst.26.1.1738] [PMID: 17633307]

[51]   Kyle JL, Harris E. Global spread and persistence of dengue. Annu Rev Microbiol 2008; 62: 71-92.
[http://dx.doi.org/10.1146/annurev.micro.62.081307.163005] [PMID: 18429680]

[52]   Lalsiamthara J, Lee JH. Virulence associated genes-deleted Salmonella Montevideo is attenuated, highly immunogenic and confers protection against virulent challenge in chickens. Front Microbiol 2016; 7: 1634.
[http://dx.doi.org/10.3389/fmicb.2016.01634] [PMID: 27785128]

[53]   Anderson RM, Spatial MAYRM. temporal, and genetic heterogeneity in host populations and the design of immunization programmes. Mathematical Medicine and Biology. J IMA 1984; 1(3): 233-66.
[PMID: 6600104]

[54]   Hay SI, Battle KE, Pigott DM, *et al.* Global mapping of infectious disease. Philos Trans R Soc Lond B Biol Sci 2013; 368(1614)20120250
[http://dx.doi.org/10.1098/rstb.2012.0250] [PMID: 23382431]

[55]   Ramsay ME, Andrews NJ, Trotter CL, Kaczmarski EB, Miller E. Herd immunity from meningococcal serogroup C conjugate vaccination in England: database analysis. BMJ 2003; 326(7385): 365-6.
[http://dx.doi.org/10.1136/bmj.326.7385.365] [PMID: 12586669]

[56]   Georgette NT. Predicting the herd immunity threshold during an outbreak: a recursive approach. PLoS One 2009; 4(1)e4168
[http://dx.doi.org/10.1371/journal.pone.0004168] [PMID: 19132101]

[57]   Metcalf CJE, Ferrari M, Graham AL, Grenfell BT. Understanding herd immunity. Trends Immunol 2015; 36(12): 753-5.
[http://dx.doi.org/10.1016/j.it.2015.10.004] [PMID: 26683689]

[58]   Plans-Rubió P. The vaccination coverage required to establish herd immunity against influenza viruses. Prev Med 2012; 55(1): 72-7.
[http://dx.doi.org/10.1016/j.ypmed.2012.02.015] [PMID: 22414740]

[59]   Dotters-Katz SK, Hughes BL. Considerations for obstetric care during the COVID-19 pandemic. Am J Perinatol 2020; 37(8): 773-9.
[http://dx.doi.org/10.1055/s-0040-1710051] [PMID: 32303077]

[60]   Clemente-Suárez VJ, Hormeño-Holgado A, Jiménez M, *et al.* Dynamics of population immunity due to the herd Effect in the COVID-19 pandemic. Vaccines (Basel) 2020; 8(2): 236.
[http://dx.doi.org/10.3390/vaccines8020236] [PMID: 32438622]

[61]   Murphy BR, Whitehead SS. Immune response to dengue virus and prospects for a vaccine. Annu Rev Immunol 2011; 29: 587-619.
[http://dx.doi.org/10.1146/annurev-immunol-031210-101315] [PMID: 21219187]

[62]   Strugnell R, Zepp F, Cunningham A, Tantawichien T. Vaccine antigens. Perspect Vaccinol 2011; 1(1): 61-88.
[http://dx.doi.org/10.1016/j.pervac.2011.05.003]

[63]   Dejnirattisai W, Wongwiwat W, Supasa S, *et al.* A new class of highly potent, broadly neutralizing antibodies isolated from viremic patients infected with dengue virus. Nat Immunol 2015; 16(2): 170-7.
[http://dx.doi.org/10.1038/ni.3058] [PMID: 25501631]

[64]   Brugha R, Keersmaekers K, Renton A, Meheus A. Genital herpes infection: a review. Int J Epidemiol 1997; 26(4): 698-709.
[http://dx.doi.org/10.1093/ije/26.4.698] [PMID: 9279600]

[65]   Baker CJ, Kasper DL. Group B streptococcal vaccines. Rev Infect Dis 1985; 7(4): 458-67.
[http://dx.doi.org/10.1093/clinids/7.4.458] [PMID: 3898306]

[66]   Nandi S, Kumar M, Manohar M, Chauhan RS. Bovine herpes virus infections in cattle. Anim Health Res Rev 2009; 10(1): 85-98.
[http://dx.doi.org/10.1017/S1466252309990028] [PMID: 19558751]

[67]   Arinaminpathy N, Lavine JS, Grenfell BT. Self-boosting vaccines and their implications for herd immunity. Proc Natl Acad Sci USA 2012; 109(49): 20154-9.
[http://dx.doi.org/10.1073/pnas.1209683109] [PMID: 23169630]

[68]   Balke I, Zeltins A. Recent advances in the use of plant virus-like particles as vaccines. Viruses 2020; 12(3): 270.
[http://dx.doi.org/10.3390/v12030270] [PMID: 32121192]

[69]   Lee KL, Twyman RM, Fiering S, Steinmetz NF. Virus-based nanoparticles as platform technologies for modern vaccines. Wiley Interdiscip Rev Nanomed Nanobiotechnol 2016; 8(4): 554-78.
[http://dx.doi.org/10.1002/wnan.1383] [PMID: 26782096]

[70]   Blanco-Lobo P, Nogales A, Rodríguez L, Martínez-Sobrido L. Novel approaches for the development of live attenuated influenza vaccines. Viruses 2019; 11(2): 190.
[http://dx.doi.org/10.3390/v11020190] [PMID: 30813325]

[71]   Rajão DS, Pérez DR. Universal vaccines and vaccine platforms to protect against influenza viruses in humans and agriculture. Front Microbiol 2018; 9: 123.
[http://dx.doi.org/10.3389/fmicb.2018.00123] [PMID: 29467737]

[72]   Sandbulte MR, Spickler AR, Zaabel PK, Roth JA. Optimal use of vaccines for control of influenza A virus in swine. Vaccines (Basel) 2015; 3(1): 22-73.
[http://dx.doi.org/10.3390/vaccines3010022] [PMID: 26344946]

[73]   Kinyanjui TM, House TA, Kiti MC, Cane PA, Nokes DJ, Medley GF. Vaccine induced herd immunity for control of respiratory syncytial virus disease in a low-income country setting. PLoS One 2015; 10(9)e0138018
[http://dx.doi.org/10.1371/journal.pone.0138018] [PMID: 26390032]

[74]   Logan J, Nederhoff D, Koch B, *et al.* 'What have you HEARD about the HERD?' Does education about local influenza vaccination coverage and herd immunity affect willingness to vaccinate? Vaccine 2018; 36(28): 4118-25.
[http://dx.doi.org/10.1016/j.vaccine.2018.05.037] [PMID: 29789242]

[75]   Masterson SG, Lobel L, Carroll MW, Wass MN, Michaelis M. Herd immunity to ebolaviruses is not a

realistic target for current vaccination strategies. Front Immunol 2018; 9: 1025.
[http://dx.doi.org/10.3389/fimmu.2018.01025] [PMID: 29867992]

[76]   Oldfield EC III, Rodier GR, Gray GC. The endemic infectious diseases of Somalia. Clin Infect Dis 1993; 16 (Suppl. 3): S132-57.
[http://dx.doi.org/10.1093/clinids/16.Supplement_3.S132] [PMID: 8443330]

[77]   van den Bosch CA. Is endemic Burkitt's lymphoma an alliance between three infections and a tumour promoter? Lancet Oncol 2004; 5(12): 738-46.
[http://dx.doi.org/10.1016/S1470-2045(04)01650-X] [PMID: 15581545]

[78]   de Pina-Costa A, Brasil P, Di Santi SM, *et al.* Malaria in Brazil: what happens outside the Amazonian endemic region. Mem Inst Oswaldo Cruz 2014; 109(5): 618-33.
[http://dx.doi.org/10.1590/0074-0276140228] [PMID: 25185003]

[79]   Gros C, Valenti R, Schneider L, Valenti K, Gros D. Containment efficiency and control strategies for the Corona pandemic costs. arXiv preprint arXiv:200400493 2020.

[80]   Prompetchara E, Ketloy C, Palaga T. Immune responses in COVID-19 and potential vaccines: Lessons learned from SARS and MERS epidemic. Asian Pac J Allergy Immunol 2020; 38(1): 1-9.
[PMID: 32105090]

[81]   Lei S, Jiang F, Su W, *et al.* Clinical characteristics and outcomes of patients undergoing surgeries during the incubation period of COVID-19 infection. E Clinical Medicine 2020; 100331

[82]   Lai CC, Shih TP, Ko WC, Tang HJ, Hsueh PR. Severe acute respiratory syndrome coronavirus 2 (SARS-CoV-2) and coronavirus disease-2019 (COVID-19): The epidemic and the challenges. Int J Antimicrob Agents 2020; 55(3)105924
[http://dx.doi.org/10.1016/j.ijantimicag.2020.105924] [PMID: 32081636]

[83]   Khamis F, Al-Zakwani I, Al Naamani H, *et al.* Clinical characteristics and outcomes of the first 63 adult patients hospitalized with COVID-19: An experience from Oman. J Infect Public Health 2020; 13(7): 906-13.
[http://dx.doi.org/10.1016/j.jiph.2020.06.002] [PMID: 32546437]

[84]   Tay MZ, Poh CM, Rénia L, MacAry PA, Ng LFP. The trinity of COVID-19: immunity, inflammation and intervention. Nat Rev Immunol 2020; 20(6): 363-74.
[http://dx.doi.org/10.1038/s41577-020-0311-8] [PMID: 32346093]

[85]   Tlaxca JL, Ellis S, Remmele RL Jr. Live attenuated and inactivated viral vaccine formulation and nasal delivery: potential and challenges. Adv Drug Deliv Rev 2015; 93: 56-78.
[http://dx.doi.org/10.1016/j.addr.2014.10.002] [PMID: 25312673]

[86]   Bhopal RS. COVID-19 zugzwang: potential public health moves towards population (herd) immunity. Public Health in Practice 2020; p. 100031.

[87]   Kissler SM, Tedijanto C, Goldstein E, Grad YH, Lipsitch M. Projecting the transmission dynamics of SARS-CoV-2 through the postpandemic period. Science 2020; 368(6493): 860-8.
[http://dx.doi.org/10.1126/science.abb5793] [PMID: 32291278]

[88]   Randolph HE, Barreiro LB. Herd Immunity: Understanding COVID-19. Immunity 2020; 52(5): 737-41.
[http://dx.doi.org/10.1016/j.immuni.2020.04.012] [PMID: 32433946]

[89]   https://www.marketwatch.com/story/these-nine-companies-are-working-on-coronavirus-treat-ents-or-vaccines-heres-where-things-stand-2020-03-06

[90]   Raoult D, Zumla A, Locatelli F, Ippolito G, Kroemer G. Coronavirus infections: Epidemiological, clinical and immunological features and hypotheses. Cell Stress 2020; 4(4): 66.

[91]   Mackay IM, Arden KE. MERS coronavirus: diagnostics, epidemiology and transmission. Virol J 2015; 12(1): 222.
[http://dx.doi.org/10.1186/s12985-015-0439-5] [PMID: 26695637]

[92] Belkaid Y, Hand TW. Role of the microbiota in immunity and inflammation. Cell 2014; 157(1): 121-41.
[http://dx.doi.org/10.1016/j.cell.2014.03.011] [PMID: 24679531]

[93] Halstead SB. Neutralization and antibody-dependent enhancement of dengue viruses. Adv Virus Res 2003; 60: 421-67.
[http://dx.doi.org/10.1016/S0065-3527(03)60011-4] [PMID: 14689700]

[94] Regan DG, Wood JG, Benevent C, *et al.* Estimating the critical immunity threshold for preventing hepatitis A outbreaks in men who have sex with men. Epidemiol Infect 2016; 144(7): 1528-37.
[http://dx.doi.org/10.1017/S0950268815002605] [PMID: 26566273]

[95] Curran JW, Lawrence DN, Jaffe H, *et al.* Acquired immunodeficiency syndrome (AIDS) associated with transfusions. N Engl J Med 1984; 310(2): 69-75.
[http://dx.doi.org/10.1056/NEJM198401123100201] [PMID: 6606780]

[96] Stull JW, Stevenson KB. Zoonotic disease risks for immunocompromised and other high-risk clients and staff: promoting safe pet ownership and contact. Vet Clin North Am Small Anim Pract 2015; 45(2): 377-392, vii.
[http://dx.doi.org/10.1016/j.cvsm.2014.11.007] [PMID: 25534535]

[97] Korhonen J, Granberg B. Sweden Backcasting, Now?—Strategic Planning for Covid-19 Mitigation in a Liberal Democracy. Sustainability 2020; 12(10): 4138.
[http://dx.doi.org/10.3390/su12104138]

[98] Irwin RE. Misinformation and de-contextualization: international media reporting on Sweden and COVID-19. Global Health 2020; 16(1): 62.
[http://dx.doi.org/10.1186/s12992-020-00588-x] [PMID: 32660503]

[99] Pattnaik B, Subramaniam S, Sanyal A, *et al.* Foot-and-mouth disease: global status and future road map for control and prevention in India. Agric Res 2012; 1(2): 132-47.
[http://dx.doi.org/10.1007/s40003-012-0012-z]

[100] Bloomfield SF, Aiello AE, Cookson B, O'Boyle C, Larson EL. The effectiveness of hand hygiene procedures in reducing the risks of infections in home and community settings including handwashing and alcohol-based hand sanitizers. Am J Infect Control 2007; 35(10): S27-64.
[http://dx.doi.org/10.1016/j.ajic.2007.07.001]

[101] Jin YH, Cai L, Cheng ZS, *et al.* A rapid advice guideline for the diagnosis and treatment of 2019 novel coronavirus (2019-nCoV) infected pneumonia (standard version). Mil Med Res 2020; 7(1): 4.
[http://dx.doi.org/10.1186/s40779-020-0233-6] [PMID: 32029004]

[102] Lloyd A, Patel N, Scott DA, Runge C, Claes C, Rose M. Cost-effectiveness of heptavalent conjugate pneumococcal vaccine (Prevenar) in Germany: considering a high-risk population and herd immunity effects. Eur J Health Econ 2008; 9(1): 7-15.
[http://dx.doi.org/10.1007/s10198-006-0013-6] [PMID: 17333089]

SUBJECT INDEX

www.ingramcontent.com/pod-product-compliance
Lightning Source LLC
Chambersburg PA
CBHW041712210326
41598CB00007B/626